WHY DIDN'T I NOTICE HER BEFORE?

A memoir about dying to live

BETH CRAMER

CONTENTS

For Todd & Noah
When I seize the moment I always want you there.

She let go.

She let go. Without a thought or a word, she let go.

She let go of the fear.

She let go of the judgments.

She let go of the confluence of opinions swarming around her head.

She let go of the committee of indecision within her.

She let go of all the "right" reasons.

Wholly and completely, without hesitation or worry, she just let go.

She didn't ask anyone for advice.

She didn't read a book on how to let go.

She didn't search the scriptures.

She just let go.

She let go of all of the memories that held her back.

She let go of all of the anxiety that kept her from moving forward.

She let go of the planning and all of the calculations about how to do it just right.

She didn't promise to let go.

She didn't journal about it.

She didn't write the projected date in her Day-Timer.

She made no public announcement and put no ad in the paper.

She didn't check the weather report or read her daily horoscope.

She just let go.

—SAFIRE ROSE

PREFACE

When I started to write *The Isa Stories,* a novel, it was influenced by several women my age living in my community who had been diagnosed with cancer. Lili, a visual artist and intellectual, was working on a series of silk screens that explored the internal landscape of her own mind. She titled it Emotional Map. At the time Lili was also going through emotional hardships: a divorce, the loss of a dog, parenting a strong-willed child, and she'd taken a significant financial hit in a Ponzi scheme.

The iconic piece in Lili's series is a self-portrait. Her hand is spread wide, pressing into her forehead as if to compress a migraine or say, "What have I done?" Her figure is an outline and within are thousands of charcoaled microbes, cells, nerve endings, and their synapses. It is an image of cells gone rogue. A few months into this project, Lili boarded a plane to visit family in Ottawa and landed with vision problems. The doctors found a large brain tumor.

Analyzing her drawings, it would be hard to deny that the tumor was reflected in her work. Was this her way of making sense of the chaos, even before its truth was revealed? Only looking back could you easily see what was most likely a premonition of her diagnosis and ultimate death. Do our subconscious minds know before illness is discovered? Can psychological variables predict subsequent disease?

After my diagnosis in September of 2017, a friend suggested I read a book written by Bernie S. Siegel, M.D. called *Love, Medicine and Miracles*. The title insinuates that recovery depends on one's willingness to believe our minds can influence the outcome. Reading deeper into the book, I latched onto this message's counterpart. If we can influence our recovery then we can influence the development of disease. The connection between my debilitating regret over an abortion I had seven years prior to my cancer diagnosis and the targeted area of my disease (the ovaries) is pretty ironic. Dr. Siegel supports the belief that the body is capable of synchronizing with our subconscious.

Dr. Siegel writes in his book, "Many documented cases show that psychological influences play a large part in determining who will develop illness. It often determines what disease will occur, and when and where it will appear," writes Siegel. He gives examples of several patients who "developed cancer in only one area that is psychologically significant to them—the target organ." One example describes a man who insisted he was pregnant and grew an enormous tumor of the urethra and prostate (the closest male equivalents of the womb) so that he looked pregnant.

Trying to make connections to my illness, I think back to a conversation I had with a psychic twenty years earlier.

My sister Mauri swore by this woman's powers. Thinking we create our own fates, I proceeded, if only for its entertainment value. The reading was done over the phone. She could not see me, nor did she have any information about me prior to the call. Prepared to spend a hundred dollars on what I expected to be folly, I curled up on my bedroom floor and listened as the psychic's assured voice told me my future.

While I did not ask questions about family, she raised the subject. "Having children will be a bit of a science experiment," she said. This was before reproductive medicine was common and motherhood was just an abstraction in my mind.

After forty-five minutes she went silent. We were not disconnected. I could hear her breath. When she spoke again, her voice had a hard edge. She informed me that since I'd agreed at the start of the session not to be told any foreboding information about my future, she could not go on.

In 1999, had I heard what inauspicious future awaited me, it would have sounded absurd, just as her vision of my experimental pregnancies did. But in 2003 one of her predictions came true in a big way. I reproduced in a lab. Scientists monitored my ovarian reserve, follicular dynamics, and biomarkers. Science hormonally altered my body to produce an egg. Did the psychic also know I would get cancer eighteen years later in September of 2017?

* * *

Writing a novel spawned by the many women around me who had recently died of cancer sparked an idea. I was desperate for any idea to cling to: my story was one I needed to let go of. Choosing to give my fictional heroine cancer made me uneasy, however. It was a big undertaking. I had to get the facts and emotions right. How could I truly understand what world she walked through with a terminal illness? Could I make her voice sound authentic? Should I just have given her anxiety and depression (that wouldn't be such a stretch) instead of cancer?

When sharing my story idea with my husband, Todd, he remarked, "That's depressing. No one wants to read about that." How could I blame him? *The Isa Stories* was sad, the subject matter unpleasant. Since I have never been close to cancer, the book would have possibly come to a halt.

When I workshopped what I called *The Isa Stories,* the first question people asked was if I had cancer. Did I say no apologetically? As I sketched my heroine, I knew she was controlling, a loving mother, and dedicated to her career as a pediatrician. It wasn't obvious to me that she was also very depressed. My readers were curious if Isa wanted to live. Apparently, readers felt an undercurrent: Isa was unhappy before her diagnosis. One day I came to the workshop and declared that Isa was dead and that I had killed her. It was too tough to write. I didn't have enough specifics. The group convinced me to resurrect her.

Perhaps my cancer began the day I put Isa on the page, seven months before our lives converged. *The Isa Stories* gave this book the kind of foreshadowing that would make me seem like a savvy storyteller. Isa and the cancer emerged inside me, slowly making their way to the surface. When I told my workshop peers I was now the one with cancer, they were shocked. All the research I needed to make the fiction believable was about to be handed to me on a silver platter.

4

1

A SPRING TERMINATION

April 15, 2009

We had a spring termination. Todd and I were at my obstetrician's office being asked if we wanted to take one last look at the ultrasound. Todd declined, and therefore, so did I. Had we looked, I might have said stop and jumped off the table. Todd might have bet on the future. Life might have been a completely different movie. What I expected to be a regretful decision became a cataclysmic event.

* * *

I had a prosperous career in film editing for twenty years. "Who lives better than us?" Todd and I would ask ourselves skiing midweek, or spending time at our home in the country. We'd made good financial choices in our early years together. We bought a loft in New York City and a house in the Hudson Valley. After Noah was born in 2004, I went right back to work, intent on making a transition into directing. The advertising world was changing, the production budgets were shrinking, and I became impatient with long hours. Regardless, I was still committed to being at the top of my game, growing my career, and being a provider. Todd was selling real estate and we had a nanny. Living in the city allowed me to be with Noah and work without too much effort. But financially, managing our loft in Soho and our house upstate would not last for long.

Renting the loft made the most sense, even though this meant I would commute ninety miles into the city for jobs, and sleep in a hotel during those times. Boxes began to replace our furniture, the loft started to echo, and four-year-old Noah crawled through cardboard tunnels. We were a sweet little family in transition.

Leaving an era behind me, I remembered the years of first independence, quick romances, and unexpected visitors at three in the morning, including the one that became my fiancé. I was the fearless, quirky, ambitious Beth who dreamed big and brought home a beautiful baby, giving everything purpose. After Noah's birth, I bet further on my future. I left the company where I'd grown my success to become a partner at another one, before going independent and seeking representation as a director. Why was I leaving the city that made having it all seem possible?

I took a break from packing to shop at CVS. The First Response tip balanced on the tumbled marble vanity as I unhappily went back to stripping my closet, feeling like I was throwing the prime of my life into a box.

Back in the bathroom, I peered down at the stick and took a step back. After years of infertility there were two red lines. My heart fluttered. Surely this was a sign, a reason for this move. I was going to raise two children in the country. I was overcome with romantic visions of two children running around my aproned legs as I conference-called clients to pitch creative treatments for my next production. It never occurred to me that I wouldn't still have it all.

How was I going to present this surprise to Todd? Should I leave it on a box and let him find it? He found the stick in the bathroom before I had a chance to decide. Looking back at that moment, I wonder if my presentation would have changed things. If I were to rewrite the script, I would have jumped into his arms while clutching the thumb grip of the pregnancy stick above my head, waving my urine-absorbed tip in victory circles. "We're having a baby!" My mistake was giving Todd an option to consider the pregnancy a choice.

Todd did take time to weigh the pros and cons, concluding that, "We have one healthy child. Why push it?" Without support for having a second child, my excitement about it couldn't grow. It never should have been contingent on one person's enthusiasm over the other's, but this was not about what restaurant we should go to, what car or property to buy, or what funds to invest in: this was a life.

How ironic, I had just finished making a documentary, *Plan B, Single Women Choosing Motherhood,* about single women consciously choosing to parent without a partner and here I imagined being faced with the same choice. Todd would not have left me, but there was a chance he would emotionally check out. He was clear

7

that having more responsibility was not something he welcomed. Meanwhile, I had no intention of giving up my career and therefore was asking a man who was not child oriented to be the primary caregiver.

I convinced myself that there would be other things to fill the empty space of a second child: more travel, directing films, less divided finances between Noah and his sibling, not having to split up who goes to which child's activities when they overlap.

When we didn't see the pregnancy through, I blamed my lack of courage and need for absolute certainty to make that decision alone. I would never forgive myself for giving up a child for no reason except that I was afraid. What followed were seven years of grief, obsession, inability to let go, difficulty concentrating, indecisiveness, and fear of making the wrong decision. There was no travel, no bigger career; Todd did not get "more" of me. There was no room for that in my broken-down soul.

One of the women in my film, *Plan B, Single Women Choosing Motherhood,* told me, "The biggest tragedy is when people talk themselves out of something when they decide it can't be possible, because if being a mother is something you want in your life, there's nothing that's going to replace it."

2

THE VISION

June 12, 2011

One year after the abortion, we were living in the Hudson Valley. Noah had just finished kindergarten and was starting first grade in the fall. I was feeling particularly well and fit. I remember telling my massage therapist that "this was going to be my year," the day before. The day before it happened.

June 11, 2011: it was a beautiful early summer night. Todd and I attended a charity auction and were in good spirits with the help of an open bar, but by the time we got to our car I was snarky, complaining about one thing or another, which frequently led to: "I wanted a second child and you didn't."

In the middle of the night Noah came into our room looking for his sleeping partner, me. I accompanied him back to bed and stayed there until dawn. I awoke, adjusted my eyes to what appeared to be a baby at the end of the bed—perfectly cherubic, about four months old, curled up chubby feet to belly, with his eyes fixed on mine. We held each other in an intense gaze that said, "We belong together." I wanted to reach out, but was frozen. Then the vision disappeared.

When I returned to my room, I formed a cocoon of covers and shut my eyes as the world spun. We were expected at my parents' beach house that afternoon, but I was afraid to move. I was like an injured victim in a horror movie who uses all their strength to grasp the phone. Struggling to reach for help, I dialed my mother. Everything felt so far away as I traveled into a new dimension. My mom answered with excited anticipation of my arrival.

"When will you be here? I'm in the car, we are all so excited." I didn't answer, but her next words were slow and filled with worry. "Beth, what's wrong?"

"Sick—I'm sick—I'm sick with regret." It's all my shaky voice could get out.

I'd been in the trenches before, having been diagnosed with a chemical imbalance at age sixteen, a feeling of ennui that lasted into my twenties. I had been in and out of therapy and was no stranger to the dark side. But this breakdown was acute. Luckily I was cognizant enough to quickly find a psychologist in my area. It was a Saturday night and I had left messages all over town. One therapist was able to see me the following day. She would end up listening to my story week after week for the next six years. My sister Mauri insisted that the vision of the baby at the bottom of the bed was me and that it was a sign of rebirth.

Besides managing my editing jobs in the city, I was on a pilgrimage to find healing. I peddled my vision and obsession to astrologers, psychics, energy healers, a divine mother, naturopaths, dream therapists, vibrational healers, acupuncturists, and specialists working in areas I'd never heard of before. I employed half of the Hudson Valley practitioners. I was shaky on my days in the editing room. I couldn't eat and lost more than ten of my ninety pounds. I shivered as if it were the middle of winter.

For months I looked at Noah and Todd, wondering how it was possible to feel so lonely in the presence of their love. Todd had to remind me to breathe. He chauffeured me to appointments. I would accompany him to the recycling station.

"I don't know what to do. I wish I could fix this."

"You could adopt," Todd responded as he drove.

All I heard was his choice of pronouns and it was singular.

One beautiful quiet night, except for the crickets, Todd and Noah slept soundly, while my mind churned. I rose and went to the kitchen pondering the meaninglessness of the ambitions I'd had just a year ago. I flipped through a design magazine and stopped at a full-page photograph of a couple and their two kids joyfully posing in front of their featured home. My heart sank. The picture was so offensive I took the magazine to the basement and pummeled it with a hammer, then ripped it to shreds. My heart ached as if nostalgic for the family I knew I would never have. Parenting and loving Noah didn't feel like enough, because I knew I would not repeat it. He would be my best work as a parent, because he would be my only. He deserved more of an experienced mother who learned with each child how to behave wisely and tenderly. Every boundary would not feel painful to create, because he wouldn't be the only one on the other side.

My three sisters made the five-hour drive from Maryland to upstate New York to be with me. They were on red alert. They kept me on the phone for five hours counseling me, telling me to hold on. When the car wheels kicked up dust on our long driveway, I was sitting on our front stoop, head in my hands. I did not know they were actually coming.

"What are you doing here?"

"We came to rescue you," they said in unison.

Todd leaned against the door frame with an impish smile, a backpack over his shoulder. He was heading into the city for the weekend to give him and us some space.

My three sisters Mauri, Karyn, and Jill and I sat on our kitchen floor for hours drinking wine and picking at sweets they'd brought from DC, neither of which I could stomach. While they were there, a neighbor showed up at my door and announced she was pregnant. They would not leave for DC until I had a prescription for Xanax. A debate arose over whether they should or shouldn't leave before seeing me actually swallow one.

Oddly, when I started driving myself to doctor's and healing appointments, an advertisement would consistently play on the radio: "If you're happy with the size of your family, make an appointment to see me to learn more about scalpel-free vasectomy or visit us online at premiere-medicalhv.com."

Around this time Todd was considering a vasectomy and polling peers who had been through the procedure.

I knew he was scared of the pain he would have to endure. Pictures of the surgery would make him woozy. This fueled something vindictive inside me. Weeks had passed since he shared his thoughts on the vasectomy and I probed about his hesitancy. It wasn't that he was having second thoughts about our family, it was that he was terrified to go under the knife. My lack of sympathy was clear, as was my opinion of his cowardice. Men have no idea how many small procedures women have to tolerate throughout their lifetimes. Didn't I recently have my feet up in stirrups, a speculum inserted into my vagina, anesthesia injected into my cervix, and a surgical instrument pry me open so a long tube connected to a suction device could draw out the fetus and the placenta?

I'm sorry I wasn't too interested in his discomfort. I took sick pleasure that his undertaking was to some extent synonymous with my calamity. He sensed I was out for revenge. I drove him to the urologist, remained in the waiting room with my arms crossed, and took my husband home with ice packs between his legs.

* * *

There was a hole I was in a hurry to fill. I didn't expect to repair the fracture, but perhaps I could rebuild. Secretly, I began researching reproductive technology and made an appointment with an endocrinologist at Cornell. I sat across the table from a world-renowned specialist and leader in the field of reproductive medicine. He held my ovarian reserve fertility test results in his hand. I caught only bits of what he was saying: "Diminished ovarian reserve"…

"poor quality"… "unlikely to conceive"… "age." My protest that I looked at least ten years younger than my age and had excellent health fell on deaf ears.

Though facts could not be disputed, the doctor offered an option. Again, the words trickled over me: "egg donor"… "shared cycle"… "shared expense"… "long waiting list." I walked out of his office and drove twenty miles over the speed limit with a thick packet of consent forms and materials explaining the egg donation process from A to Z. I should have accepted my wrong turn off Route 17 as an omen. The street sign where I made the U-turn said CRAMER'S COURT AND BELOW IT DEAD END.

As conflicted, ambivalent, scared, and alone as I was in my quest, I could not stop. Step by step, I made my way over many hurdles. My spirit was tenacious. I was its marionette, obeying its command. Imagining myself working alongside "god" to create a new reality. It was the most narcissistic I had ever been. Since Todd had gotten his vasectomy, I was going to have to persuade him to have his sperm aspirated. They would still be plentiful, healthy, and easy to retrieve.

I am, fundamentally, a practical person. Nothing in my life had prepared me for this level of crazy. I truly believed I would stumble off the earth into an abyss of nothingness without another child to hold me. I also feared another child could jeopardize the family I had. Todd was opposed to another child and Noah liked being the only. However, if I didn't do this, I also knew I would be managing regret the rest of my life. Though my therapist told me that this obsession was a violent action toward myself, I could not stop.

* * *

It is an arduous process finding an egg donor and following the strict schedule necessary to create a child. Months of secrecy and filling out documents ensued. The donor they paired me with seemed perfect. She was a college student, a Buddhist, she exercised, was attractive, and taller than me. My child would not have to worry about height or depression.

Following a match I needed to do what is called a "prep cycle" to make sure my ovarian lining responded to medication and so the donor and I could synchronize our cycles. The prep cycle should last twenty-one days. It took me one hundred and eighty-nine. Nine prep cycles and not because I wasn't responding to the medication. Every morning I would question my motives, my commitment to this dream, and the toll it was taking on my relationship with Todd. I was acting out of desperation not joy, yet I would start one prep cycle and quit after three days, each time letting myself go a bit further until calling it off. On my ninth try, I got through the full twenty-one days of preparation, but did not show up for my final ultrasound and blood work. I was reliving the abortion.

Each cycle required that I give myself intramuscular injections of Lupron, FSH, HCG, and hormones galore. I prepared the needles and shot up on my own without help. My therapist pointed out that I was basically a cutter, inflicting self-harm on myself.

Her words sank in as I was making my way upstairs to administer another shot. I sat in the middle of the stairs and cried. Yes, I yearned for that second child, the one I'd lost, but I was punishing myself for it. I wanted to have another chance to parent and this was my best option, but I was sabotaging my chances.

Besides stabbing myself daily with one-and-a-half-inch needles, raiding my bank account, and keeping secrets, I was spending an enormous amount of time preoccupied with this experiment. Genetic screening, blood tests on a weekly basis, deadlines, coordinating: it was sheer insanity. I was being torn apart by ambivalence and thunderclouds of "what ifs." Regardless, I kept moving forward. Don't get me wrong, there is no doubt I had a desire for this child—this was not magical thinking—but there was some other factor I still don't understand driving my anxiety to incredibly strong heights. Someone was calling to be in the family, but it was in direct conflict with another voice. Something was holding me back even when I was certain I wanted to move forward. What was my ambivalence serving? Is it possible cancer was always in the background?

Hours would go by. I could not read with any focus or hold a conversation. I had only one thought in my head at all times: I have to fix this. But I was in a battle with shame and fear, a gruesome war with no end in sight. My thoughts were obsessive; I feared any future without Noah or another child in it. I would walk into Noah's room and ache looking at his collections of key chains, stones, and international currency on the floor in neat piles. He would go off and have another life soon. Noah was only six at the time.

There was no rational reason for my actions. I did not think I deserved punishment and yet it was happening. This is what mental illness looks like. I didn't want it any more than I wanted cancer.

Finally, I had to choose one path or the other. In 2014, two years after I'd met with my reproductive endocrinologist and considered using an egg donor, I followed through with an embryo transfer. The day of the transfer Todd and I sat across from each other in the waiting room at Cornell surrounded by young couples holding hands and giggling. I started crying. The receptionist got up and handed me a box of tissues. My tears didn't seem like the right emotion for this occasion and she was afraid I would scare the other patients. What was playing through my headphones only amplified my tears: the song I referred to as my second baby anthem, "A Thousand Years" by Christina Perri summed up everything I felt about my relationship to that soul, the one I'd lost, and the one waiting.

I have died every day waiting for you
Darling, don't be afraid
I have loved you
For a thousand years
I'll love you for a thousand more
Time stands still

Beauty in all she is

I will be brave
I will not let anything take away
What's standing in front of me
Every breath
Every hour has come to this
One step closer

After the transfer it was suggested that I rest on my back in the recovery room for at least an hour. When they called Todd into my cubical ten minutes after my procedure, I told him we could go. We were going to be late for dinner. Remembering that my doctor had told me nothing I did after the transfer could affect the outcome. He said heroin addicts get pregnant every day. I decided waiting the full hour was unnecessary. Todd had had more than a few reservations about my behavior recently. He had every right to. I did not act like a woman wanting to be pregnant. I acted like I was going to prison. It was very awkward knowing in the back of my mind that I was still uncertain about what the hell I was doing. My chance had been seven years earlier, when so much convincing was unnecessary and I'd had an abortion instead.

The transfer was unsuccessful and we decided to freeze the other two embryos. My anxiety did not abate and Todd questioned my ability to parent at all. What if I did go off the deep end and he was left raising two children?

* * *

On bad days, I would intend to go for a run, but sit in my car instead with the key in the ignition as nervous as a drug addict suffering from withdrawal. I would call my mom in these moments: "Me again, same time different day, same problem, same anxiety, same I'm not going to take in anything you tell me, but thank you for listening." One day—I'll never forget it, because it sounded so harsh coming from this gentle woman—my mother said, "You might as well have cancer."

3

THE ECLIPSE

August 17–23, 2017

"There's going to be a solar eclipse, can we go see it?" Noah's sixth grade science teacher had sparked his imagination.

"Of course," I blurt out.

"We have to be in the umbra; that's where the sun will be completely blocked," Noah says with enthusiasm. "It's called totality. We want that. We don't want to be in the penumbra, that's only partial."

"Carpe diem! We're going to see the eclipse. Road trip!" I commit without information as my husband shakes his head, letting me know he won't be joining us. I have taken Noah on a trip to Guatemala by myself. I can do this.

The travel map I hang in my head has color-coded push-pins marking our stops between Delaware and Nashville, including the return trip to New York. The car is loaded with video equipment including a newly purchased drone. Noah wants to be a director and editor just like his mother and here is a teaching opportunity. This trip gives us a script with a clear beginning, middle, and end.

OPENING SCENE:

EXT. COASTAL HIGHWAY—MORNING
Aerial shot tracking Mini Cooper traveling from Delaware toward Virginia Beach making its way to Nashville, Tennessee.

INT. CAR
We rock to the first song on our road trip soundtrack. We head-bang to the music. Sun-kissed faces and exuberant smiles mix with serious determination.

Noah takes video of the cars passing on the highway before popping headphones in and switching over to downloaded episodes of *Family Guy* on his iPad. Though I see where we are headed, I keep my eyes on the road. I turn on NPR at a reasonable level. Noah reaches over and turns it down. An ongoing arm-wrestling tournament ensues.

Traveling west on I-40 feels epic. Every time I pass this iconic road sign, I feel accomplished. My son's face may be trained on an iPad, but I motor on, holding onto expectations for the both of us, and my bragging rights.

Red flashing neon signs warn: SOLAR ECLIPSE AUGUST 21ST PLAN AHEAD EXPECT DELAYS. We are really doing this. Chapel Hill, North Carolina completes the first leg. Great, happy. Noah has a fantastic conversation with a Kenyan Uber driver who shares his name. We have dinner with my nephew, Sam, his cousin. Second leg: Asheville, North Carolina, a cool hippie-turned-hipster community with its coffee houses, secondhand shops, farm-to-table restaurants, and taco shacks. This is the Asheville I want to explore, but the first evening Noah wants to explore the hotel room with its flat-screen TV, WiFi, and pillow-top mattress that makes it feel as though he is sleeping in a cloud.

After six hours in the car followed by a tour of the Biltmore Estate, where Noah once again redeems himself as my ideal travel companion, I allow him to settle in for the night. Venturing out alone to bring back a Mexican feast is disappointing, but the glass of sauvignon blanc at the bar helps ease the letdown. Returning to the hotel bar before heading up to the room softens it more.

Noah wakes with renewed energy for chocolate-chip pancakes and bacon. The top of act two: the promise of the premise. It's when the setup is finished, and the characters have fun; it's the trailer moments. Willing to navigate with no Yelp advice we find the best breakfast spot in Asheville. We use our wait time to wander the farmer's market, filling our bag with anything Noah desires. Noah becomes a foodie and his appreciation for the bounty fills my soul. These are the moments I treasure.

Wanting to hold onto our joy in Asheville I sponta-neously declare we will spend another night. Every hotel within the area including ours is booked; they are coming in droves for the eclipse.

Nashville, Tennessee, music city, the land of Elvis and Dolly, strip clubs and bars. We drive through without leav-ing the car. Noah takes some fine pictures from the win-dow, but the seedy side of Nashville holds no allure for us.

Before giving up on Nashville, however, we find an upscale neighborhood with hip restaurants and boutiques where we stumble across a Frye shoe store. With no intention of buying anything, I find myself opening the heavy door to boots: tall, ankle, Western, and a pair of tanned leather ankle-high boots with a platform heel, vintage but modern. Noah entertains himself by hiding behind the displays, but becomes impatient. I consider my round-trip drive from New York to Nashville, my dedication to my son having this experience, all my planning, my courage for doing it alone without my husband, and how thrifty I've been over the past few years. Don't I deserve these boots? Three hundred and fifty-eight dollars poorer, and with a bit of shame, I leave the store.

The final destination is a ranch outside of Nashville and it does not disappoint. Noah is in awe of the room with its Western décor complete with taxidermy above the bed, the swimming pool, and the little dog that belongs to the property. It takes me a while to figure out the WiFi password, but once we get that going he sits back to watch a marathon of *Riverdale*.

The owner recommends a Mexican restaurant down the road so I go for takeout, convincing myself that it's okay for Noah and me to have individual experiences while sharing space and a common goal. Plus this gives me an opportunity to stop at the deli to pick up a six-pack of Corona. I don't usually drink beer, but I am in the middle of nowhere and I need to fuel my enthusiasm and idealism. I need this experience to be intoxicating.

Act Three: Bad Guys Close In. The night before the eclipse I learn we are not in the path of totality. We need to drive at least forty minutes to be inside the umbra. There is no choice but to set a new coordinate. Next morning our wheels speed northwest, chasing the eclipse like storm trackers. With my anxiety mounting and Noah's frustration over my many U-turns, much is at stake.

Finally I pull into an empty elementary school parking lot. There is not a patch of shade to cool us from what feels like 140 degrees Fahrenheit. Noah doesn't want to leave the air-conditioned car. The car has a skylight so we can watch the approach and jump out of the car for the main event. I set up our chairs, come back for Noah, but he's not budging.

"The eclipse is starting. Don't you want to set up?"

"I can see it through the skylight. I'll get out when it's time."

"How will you know? You're looking at the iPad."

"Mom!"

I mope away, crestfallen. Why is he resisting? Am I no longer good company? Is the show he is watching that engrossing? We drove sixteen hours to see this. It was his idea that led us here and it was a good one. I blame his iPad. Then I blame myself for being overly zealous. I could have made Asheville our destination; it also is in direct line of the eclipse and five hours closer to home! I'm sure I thought the more mileage we traveled the more stories we would have, the more we could boast.

Determined to not let Noah burst what's left of my deflated bubble, I don my headphones, cue up the playlist I created specifically for the eclipse, and take to my viewing spot. Texts come through from Todd in New York enjoying a partial eclipse with friends and strangers. The pictures show them sharing eclipse glasses, flasks, and a joint. Why is he having all the fun? He didn't drive across country to catch the full eclipse.

He drove five minutes up the mountain from our home.

I dig my toes into the grass and find a song to help access my inner child. Venom rises from my gut; I'm fearful of my rage and my expectations. This is Noah's experience, too, but I don't want him to look back with regret. I flail my arms in the car's direction mouthing, "It's time, you're going to miss it!" Pulling the car door open, I swoop in as if to catch my prey. "What are you doing? We came all this way. Aren't you going to come see it with me?"

"It's too hot, I can see it through the skylight. I can see everything," Noah says, but doesn't look up.

"But this is supposed to be a shared experience."

Returning to my station, I raise my music to peak. A shadow hangs over me, not the eclipse; it's Noah. Though he has decided to join me, it's obvious it is only to appease. "Go back to the car," I say. "Make sure to look up every once in a while and wear the glasses. I love you."

Totality will last two minutes and thirty-seven seconds. The moon cutting across the sun is more spectacular than full darkness. Did I spend entirely too much time planning this moment? The eclipse itself may have been the impetus, but there has to be a deeper significance.

* * *

Back at the ranch we jump in the pool. The eclipse glasses sit on the lounge chair. I grab a pair, put them on, and toss the second pair to Noah who is relaxing on a pool float. Our equilibrium now balanced, we are playful with each other. The worst is over. I ask if I can take his picture floating on the raft looking up at the sky wearing the glasses.

"This," I say, "is where we saw the eclipse. This is how we will always remember it and we will never, ever mention the elementary school parking lot."

"I'm a jerk. I don't know what I was thinking. Sorry I let you down."

"It's okay, Noah. Let's delete that part. In this pool, just as we are now, is how we saw it. Forget the rest." Lying on those rafts, believing our lie; that was the picture I posted on Facebook. In that moment we rewrote the finale.

* * *

It was August 21, 2017 when we returned home. Three weeks later I would learn I had driven nine hundred miles not knowing I had stage 4 ovarian cancer. The eclipse wasn't the goal; it was our metaphor, our theme. Together we made a plan, realized a dream, and said yes to life.

* * *

FINAL IMAGE THREE MONTHS LATER— AFTER DIAGNOSIS

INT. HOME—DAY

Me lying on the couch, a cancer patient with a cue ball head under a knitted beanie, wrapped in a blanket replaying a video of Noah and me setting out on our journey, bobbing our heads to the music. The youthful woman in the driver's seat mesmerizes me with her long golden-brown hair framing her face in a soft wave. She radiates all the love in the world for the boy next to her. She exudes a can-do attitude and a rock-and-roll spirit. Why didn't I notice her before?

4

CANCER ALL MINE

September 10–15, 2017

It is September tenth and I can feel a chill in my bones. The expired Zoloft in my medicine cabinet reminds me of how my anxiety can get out of control. I swallow fifty milligrams.

Three years ago we had an exchange student come live with us for the school year. Todd's enthusiasm around this idea was surprising, as he did not share my longing for more noise in our house. My sensible husband had found a quick Band-Aid to stop my emotions from leaking into another school year and to quiet the unfinished debate over our family's size. Noah would get an older brother, and I could pretend I had two children for one year. I have to admit it was a clever and loving gesture. The boy from Germany was not a great fit, partially because I was still at the height of my mourning and compulsive quest to fill the hole. There was no desire on my part to host again.

* * *

Todd had received an email from AFS, the international exchange program, again in 2017. He asked me if I would host again. Call it a whim or a premonition, but I gave an enthusiastic yes. Something about this particular boy, Tom, was part of a divine plan that would start to unfold one week after his arrival.

September 11, 2017, I wake in the middle of the night with indigestion that I hope is not a heart attack. In the morning I call my sister Karyn, whose underactive thyroid causes her heartburn. She verifies my condition and rattles off a few questions regarding my bowels.

"Do you have a gastroenterologist?"

"No."

"Can you get a referral to see one?"

"I think so. Also I've had this weird lump in my abdomen I've been meaning to check out."

"Why haven't you seen a doctor?"

"It's one of those things that will go away on its own. It's probably a stubborn feces in my descending colon."

She pauses. When she speaks again her voice sounds stern. "Make an appointment with a gastroenterologist today. Call and get a referral."

Getting a fast appointment is never so easy. The heartburn has subsided by the time I get to the doctor's that early afternoon. I consider leaving, but I know my sister and Todd would be mad if I complained of heartburn again. Before I have a chance to pick up a magazine my name is called.

I am downright cheery as I follow a nurse practitioner to an examination room. I banter along the way like it's our first date. "I didn't even have time to pick a magazine. Your office is awesome. I've already written your review."

"So what brings you in?"

"It's kind of stupid, but heartburn. Could taking expired Zoloft cause that?"

"I don't know, but I can give you something to relieve the heartburn."

The nurse practitioner leaves the room and reappears with an armful of Prilosec samples. She dumps them on the chair next to me and writes me a prescription for more. Assuming my case is closed she starts to leave. "Wait, one more thing. Can you take a look at this bump and tell me what it is?"

"A bump?"

"A bump or lump. It's been there a while. Maybe a feces that needs to loosen?"

"Come sit on the table for me."

I sit on the edge of the medical table and lean back. "It's here." I point to my pelvis.

She touches the spot and pulls her hand back as if scorched. Her smile disappears. Her prescription pad flies out, she scribbles something on it, and hands me the slip like it's a relay race. I read it: "Abdominal CT scan," and on top "STAT."

The women at reception who signed me in at a leisurely pace are now scurrying to get my CT scan pre-approved by insurance and making urgent phone calls to the nearest radiology centers. The first wave of panic washes over me. "I will never do anything I don't want to again," I tell myself as I run to my car.

I make the three-minute drive to the closest radiology center in Kingston, NY. Although the address is correct, the building appears condemned. People enter below the worn radiology signage as I sit in my car and deliberate. Tentatively, I lock my doors and enter the office. The crowded waiting room assures me this is the place. The interior is clean so with faith and the prescription tight between my forefinger and thumb, I saddle up to the registrar and slide it in front of her as if I'm dealing cards at a casino. "Do you have an appointment?" she asks without looking up.

"My doctor's office should have called to say I was coming."

"You have to sign in at the kiosk if you don't have an appointment," the woman says.

"But look, the prescription says STAT."

"Do you have pre-approval?" She looks up at me; her expression turns to pity. Insurance, ugh. I could be dying, blood pooling around me and I would still have to wait for pre-approval to get a Band-Aid. I sit. I wait. "Ms. Cramer?" So being STAT does mean I am going to jump the line.

My blood is taken and I am ushered to another small waiting room where I join a group of seniors drinking Big Gulps. A nurse hands me the Big Gulp; the liquid resembles thinned-out Elmer's Glue. She instructs me to drink the thirty-two ounces before two o'clock. This means Noah is going to be home from school before me. As I sit here for an hour learning new medical terms, new tastes, and new things to hate, it dawns on me: this CT scan is the material I need for my *Isa Stories.*

While I am lying horizontal on a conveyer belt pushing me back and forth through a tube, Todd is in New York City finalizing the sale of our loft that we had been renting out since relocating to New Paltz. We intend to use the money to pay off our credit cards and for nonessentials such as vacations. How do I tell Todd the only trip we most likely will take with this money is to the hospital?

My ride home is filled with dread over how I am going to greet Noah. This boy is telepathic when it comes to reading me. I hope the dog won't notice. Dogs always know. They don't need to be told. I think, goddamn it, how can I face the dog?

My cell phone rings as I am making Noah a snack and casually discussing the day. I hurry into the bathroom as soon as I hear the nurse's voice. "They found something very concerning on your CT scan, very concerning. You have to come in tomorrow to see an oncologist and you must bring your husband. Dr. Laghari is going to China the next day, but he's coming in just for you. This is very serious. It's likely cancer."

Noah is honing in on my monosyllabic responses: "Really?" "No," "No way," and "What?"

* * *

It is Tuesday, September 12, my sisters and I are to meet in Bethany Beach, Delaware to celebrate my dad's eighty-fifth birthday in three days, and I am about to ruin the occasion.

Stepping back into the kitchen, I meet Noah's suspicious glare. "Who was that? What was that about?"

"It's not important."

"Why aren't you telling me the truth?"

"I was just scheduling an appointment."

"For what? What's wrong?"

"Nothing, Noah. It's a routine appointment. I was confirming it."

Noah simmers with anger and runs upstairs. For once I am grateful he does because this gives me an opportunity to go out to the car and call Karyn. Todd is not home yet. If I call him while he is driving that could be dangerous. Karyn answers. "It's not heartburn. The gastro sent me for a CT scan. I don't think that bump was a feces. They found something, they don't know what, but it is very concerning."

Todd arrives home relieved that the burden of managing our loft is over and that the sale went smoothly. We should be celebrating. "Did you get to see a doctor?" he asks as he takes a beer from the refrigerator.

"I saw a nurse practitioner."

"And?"

"She sent me for a CT scan."

"For heartburn?"

"No, for a lump they found in my pelvis."

"Wait. Back up."

"They're very concerned by what they found. We have to go see an oncologist tomorrow morning. The doctor's coming in just for me before going to a conference in China. They want you to come with me."

"Of course. What time?"

"Ten."

"Where?"

"Kingston. I have to see an oncologist, Todd. I had to look that up just to see what they specialize in. Cancer, that's what an oncologist is for."

Did Todd know what an oncologist does or, like me, has he never thought of needing one? Nothing more is said about the meeting or our fear. As a rule we don't talk about things in the abstract, we wait for confirmation. So with neither of us exposing any vulnerability the night passes.

*　*　*

Wednesday, September 13, at ten o'clock, Todd and I walk into the oncologist's office like two innocent people about to be charged with a criminal offence. My iPhone's Voice Memos app is recording before we step into the examination room. Whatever we are about to hear I get the sense we will need to hear it again and I have to admit it would be good material for *The Isa Stories*. The first ten minutes, before the doctor enters, the only thing on the recording is the air-conditioning's hiss. We both flinch when the door opens.

"Hi, Ms. Cramer. How are you? Dr. Laghari."

"Nice to meet you, thank you for coming in today." I sound like I'm here to interview him.

"So how long have you been symptomatic?"

"I haven't. I mean there is a lump in my pelvis."

He looks carefully at my chart. I wonder why he doesn't want to touch my lump.

"Do you have any trouble moving your bowels?"

"No."

"Indigestion, anything like that?"

"Not really," I answer.

"But pretty severe the last few nights. She couldn't sleep and a lot of pain right in the sternum," Todd interjects.

"Bloating sensation?"

"No."

"Big belly, you know?" Dr. Laghari asks.

"Well, my belly has been distended for…" Uh-oh.

Dr. Laghari continues, "You feeling heavy down there?"

I can only assume what "down there" means. "No."

"Any nausea? Vomiting?"

"No."

"Appetite has decreased?"

"Just the last day."

"What about urination? It's pressing on the bladder. You don't feel any frequency during the night?"

"No." What the hell is pressing on my bladder?

"Medically any problems?"

"No."

"Smoking? Drinking?"

"I drink wine."

"Smoking? No?" I shake my head. "Any family history of any cancer?"

"No."

"Any kids?"

"Yes. One son. He's thirteen."

"Did anyone explain to you about the CT scan? Looking at it, it looks like you have an ovarian tumor. It's big. Ovarian tumor." Dr. Laghari's Indian accent is clear enough, but I don't understand what he is saying. He flips over the report and sketches what appears to be a bull with horns. It takes a moment to recognize the fallopian tubes. I wish I had paid attention in anatomy class. How am I even standing? I am looking over Dr. Laghari's shoulder as if he is showing me architectural plans.

"So they are seeing some lymph nodes in the back. The biggest one is one-point-five centimeters beneath the bowel. And then what you are feeling on the right side, there is a four-point-one centimeter tumor. Now in the pelvis—"

"What!? There's more?"

"There is a large tumor there. It's big. It has to come out. It's fourteen centimeters. They can't see the ovaries. You have to go for surgery."

I experience a head rush, I see stars and a flashback. For many, many months I walked around with a big belly on my petite frame. Friends and family laughed at how adorable I looked even in my bikini, as if I were pregnant or gaining weight. Assuming that this was fat storage in the abdomen, indicating menopause, I didn't think much of it except that it was annoying. Now I realize my belly was not carrying a baby or fat, but a fourteen-centimeter tumor blocking my ovaries.

"They are going to remove the big mass, remove the uterus, ovaries, fallopian tubes, all of it. They call it debulking." I don't pause to consider this procedure's unfortunate name. "After that you're going to need chemotherapy."

I gasp. Todd bows his head, we both cry. I want to clasp my hands over my ears. It's unthinkable.

"You have to—you have to," he says, "it's very aggressive." Between my sobs, as if I didn't hear him, he repeats, "It's very advanced. I'm going to order a CT scan of the chest."

As I recall the unexplained sore throats I've had over the past year and that strange knob I felt in my neck a week ago, I correct him, "CT scans of the neck and chest." I raise my head to the ceiling, "Oh my god. Noah."

Todd grabs my hand. "One step at a time."

Dr. Laghari goes over some logistics with the nurse. Did the nurse already know my results when she led me into the exam room? How I must have changed during that time: hunched over, pale, and weight dripping off my body.

"We will request for it STAT," Dr. Laghari tells me.

"Yup," I say as if I'm an old pro.

"What does that stand for?" Todd asks.

Dr. Laghari and the nurse speak in unison. "Right away, immediately." They laugh unexpectedly.

"I know, but I hear it all the time and never know where it comes from," Todd continues.

Dr. Laghari actually hoots. "I don't know."

"I don't know actually," the nurse also admits.

"Okay, nobody knows. I was just wondering its origin," Todd says.

Dr. Laghari thinks about this. "It's one of those strange things. Actually let's find out." Is he really going to the computer and typing STAT into his search engine? I see his eyes scanning the results. "Nothing is coming up. Oh well. Interesting question though." As an afterthought Laghari looks at me and says, "I'll write you a prescription for Ativan. You'll need it. You can take up to four milligrams a day.

On our way out of the office I'm handed a spiral organizer to log my medical notes and appointment dates. My cancer is official. I am on my way back to radiology, but this time with a witness to this absurdity. Todd follows my directions to the radiology center, but stops before pulling into the lot. "Are you sure this is it? What's the address?"

"This is it."

"I don't see a sign."

"I was here yesterday. Believe me, it's the place." Still skeptical Todd follows me in. "I'm back," I tell the receptionist. This time she doesn't ask me to sign in at the kiosk.

* * *

I did this, I tell myself. Todd's eyes are fixed on the road. I don't dare let my thoughts spill out. I know my diagnosis is an intervention by something greater than myself. I had punished myself for years, I ran out of ideas on how to. I gave up trying to have another child and chose to manage regret. I gave up on myself with that one loss. My battle wasn't ceasing and the gods were getting restless, bored with my one story. I was stuck on one idea with no resolution.

Cancer was suddenly braided into my novel, but moreover it gave me a resolution to my story: the second pregnancy story. I never would have thought of this as a resolution, but it's kind of brilliant. And while it is replacing one ache with another, it's easy to live with cancer as long as you present healthy and have enough energy to get through the day. It's a vacation from anxiety. Cancer arrived as an antidote to living every day in fear. Even with antidepressants I battled my anxiety. I was in overtime and could hear the buzzer sound, "Cancer! Game over. If you won't let go of your second-child story, here is something that will." At this point I had no choice but to say, "Welcome, baby cancer."

* * *

While the pasta water reaches a boil, I lean over the kitchen counter and I feel it: the ache in my back, the sore throat, my bloated belly. I haven't eaten in days. Why do all the symptoms want to make themselves known today? Ovarian cancer is rare. It is called the silent killer. That is one scary term. Most people such as myself have no warning signs. I learned that it often occurs sporadically in people with no family history of the condition. What I find shocking is that it's almost never found at an early stage and once found it has already spread to other organs and difficult to treat.

A mammogram can detected breast cancer before a doctor can feel it. Women can check for lumps by placing your left hand on your hip and reach with your right hand to feel in the left armpit. Simply by checking both sides for lumps or thickenings above and below your collarbone can signal a warning.

Have you ever been told to look for signs of ovarian cancer or recognize the symptoms? According to the American Cancer Society, currently there are no reliable screening tests for ovarian cancer. While some women diagnosed with ovarian cancer have elevated levels of the CA 125 protein, the associated blood test is not accurate enough for ovarian cancer screening, as many noncancerous conditions can increase the CA 125 level. For that reason, no major medical or professional organization recommends the routine use of the CA 125 blood test to screen for ovarian cancer in women at average risk. When I was diagnosed my CA 125 value was at 231 units/ml outside the standard range of 0–35 units/ml. It would have been okay with me to have taken the test and found out it was wrong, but I had the option to find out if it was right.

What are the symptoms of ovarian cancer anyway? Constipation, unusual abdominal pain, abdominal or pelvic pressure or bloating, feeling extremely full after meals, weight gain or loss, constipation or diarrhea, nausea, flatulence, back pain, and fatigue. Really? Those are the symptoms of being a woman. Irritable bowel syndrome—talk amongst yourselves. Apparently I mistook abnormal ovarian cells gone rogue that created tumors with a chronic, functional gastrointestinal disorder. Oh well.

Dr. Laghari's flight leaves in a few hours, but once again he is back in his office for me. "I'm sorry, the cancer has metastasized." I don't know exactly what that means, but I know it's not good. If it was advanced disease yesterday, what is it today? That swollen gland I felt last week? Yup. Tumor. Fast dividing cancer cells also occupy my chest. Stage 4, advanced. Debulking has to wait. Three cycles of chemotherapy first, surgery, then three cycles of chemotherapy after. It doesn't matter that I answer "no" to every question on the medical information form: no illness, no conditions, no family history.

* * *

At two o'clock on Wednesday, September 13, after our meeting with Dr. Laghari, I call Karyn with the news that I have stage 4 cancer. "Hi. Where are you?" I ask casually when she picks up her phone at Nordstrom Rack, shopping with friends. "I'll call you later," I say.

"Tell me now. Just wait a second; let me get to a quiet place." Sitting on the floor in the corner of Nordstrom

38

Rack, she braces herself for what turns out to be what she calls the most shocking news she ever had in her whole life. Cancer is far out of our experience as a family.

Karyn will call Mauri and I will call Jill. Mauri is in Colorado working, and collapses to the ground when she hears the news. "She can't possibly have cancer, cancer doesn't run in our family, mental illness does." Jill, at her home in DC, sinks to the floor and wonders, "Why not me?"

I can't tell my mom, certainly not when she is alone. We devise a plan: Karyn and Jill will surprise Mom at the beach the day before we'd planned. A half hour after they arrive I will call. Mom answers all chipper.

"Mom, I'm not going to be able to come."

Mom's first thought is that Noah is not doing very well or that I am depressed. I remember my "sick with regret" phone call seven years ago. She tried to counsel me and promised I would recover, but this is stage 4 cancer and there will be no promises.

Mom fell silent. It doesn't matter what I said to soften it, all she heard was stage 4 ovarian cancer. At that moment, she sounded so far away, like she left her body. "This is not my life," Mom says. "This is not yours."

* * *

She is up all night as my father sleeps heavily beside her. She will have to be strong enough to tell Dad the news in the morning. He is already worried about everything under the sun. He has been consumed the entire summer with fears of a flood that might damage the house. Mom has him sit in a chair with Karyn and Jill beside him. His reaction is utter shock. He shakes so badly. He won't say anything. "Mike, it's going to be okay," Mom says and then over and over again, "This is the flood. This is the flood."

From that moment on, Mom and my sisters can't do things fast enough. They don't know what to do, but no matter what they plan to be with me in New York or wherever I get treatment. Picture air traffic controllers at a major airport hub the day before Thanksgiving. Every operator is calling their resources, reaching out to hospitals and sharing their results.

It is as if their knowledge of my disease broke the levees. I have been living with a fourteen-centimeter tumor in my belly that has metastasized to my chest and neck for probably over a year. My sisters and mom work a crisis hotline while Todd and I sit in our kitchen downing glasses of wine. Tomorrow afternoon we are heading to Albany Memorial Hospital to see a surgeon. Noah and our exchange student, Tom, play Xbox in the library and I don't stop them after four hours.

Meanwhile I add up the signs leading to this reality. One, I was writing a book about a woman with cancer. Two, my cancer is not genetic, but grew from my ovaries— the organ of my obsession, starting with the abortion and leading to assisted reproductive technology. Three, Tom entered our home at the exact time Noah could use a companion and his presence would add life to our house should I need to be somewhere else for treatment. It is as if an angel was sent to help distract him.

* * *

An hour before Todd and I are about to leave for Albany, a call comes from Mauri. She has booked me on a four o'clock flight out of New York to DC. There is a renowned gynecological surgeon at Johns Hopkins who is making time to see me the next morning.

I quickly throw a few clothes into a carry-on and wait outside for Todd. Todd finds me with my small bag at my feet and my head in my hands, sobbing. I am leaving him, Noah, and all that I consider home. I might not return. Todd and I both accept this intervention without discussion, we know Albany would never do, it is not even a nationally ranked cancer center. Between Sloan Kettering (ranked second) and Johns Hopkins (ranked six) only one is the logical choice. Receiving treatment where my three sisters and mother can care for me without uprooting them from their lives makes the most sense for everyone, everyone but me.

Todd is so contained on our race to the airport I don't know if he is in shock, feeling abandoned, or inconvenienced. "I'm just trying to get you to the airport on time."

It's true I am dangerously close to missing the flight. In the passenger seat I stew with anger at his silence, even though I recognize his process: not to process. It is Todd being left behind to manage and maintain the machine; I'm relying on him for it not to break down.

The car screeches in front of terminal B and I dash. I have my ticket but of course I can't predict airport security. At the checkpoint, I step into the *Star Trek* portal, arms up in surrender as it encircles my body. "Please, God, please, God, hurry up."

"Step aside, ma'am. Are you wearing any metal?" asks an official. He whips out his laser and paints my body with it. He hands me over to a female agent who pats me down. They both look perplexed.

The woman can't find anything on me, but points to the monitor. Distinctly displayed on the monitor is a suspicious mass about two inches long on my right pelvis. It looks like I am hiding an explosive. "That's where my tumor is," I say, shocked. The agents silently agree no one would make up a story like this and let me go. If only I had flown in the last year, a simple walk through an airport scanner could have saved my life.

A patronizing voice announces, "Final boarding call for gate twenty-four." My first movie moment is about to premiere as I yell, "Wait, wait! Hold the plane! I have cancer!"

5

HOMECOMING

September 15, 2017

I stepped off the plane in my worn blue jeans, unintentionally ripped at the knee, and my much loved, thinning cashmere sweater I refer to as Binky. My self-esteem started to wane once I handed over my ticket at the gate. By the time we touch down in Maryland my power will be submerged. I left New York a strong, persuasive, outspoken mother and wife, but will arrive in Maryland an underclassman, still finding my voice among three older sisters. Even my carry-on bag feels insignificant. I recall my therapist telling me I need to take up more space. I weave easily around the travelers and straight into the arms of my mom and three sisters: Mauri the oldest, Karyn the second oldest, Jill the third. I am the baby.

Growing up, Mom guaranteed us that we would never find best friends outside our clan. As our moniker, "the Cramer girls," suggests, we are an exclusive bunch.

I am the only sister not living in Maryland, but I am always on the text thread to meet for coffee in twenty minutes. Knowing I am three hundred miles from their Starbucks doesn't stop them from including me. This is not an oversight, but a central theme to our family dynamics, both the constructive and destructive ways we see ourselves as individuals and as a part of the whole. Whenever I get these texts, I always get phantom limb pain.

I can't help but think of *Little Women,* the four sisters and their tight bonds, guided by their mother, by faith, and their passage of childhood to womanhood. I imagine "the Cramer girls" as "the March girls"; in both stories it is Beth, the quiet sister, the one not willing to conform to social conventions, that teeters on the brink of death.

It is strange to do something drastically different than my sisters, for instance, get cancer. Before my transgression, "the Cramer girls" were the luckiest people alive, according to witnesses. I feel like I just found out I was adopted.

On arrival in Maryland my sisters shower me with gifts. My oldest sister, Mauri, presents a beautiful, long, open-front cashmere sweater that makes every body wish they had cancer; Karyn gives me four incredibly soft T-shirts; Jill supplies me with a handful of humorous books; and Mom gives me a tall mug that says, "I get up, I walk, I fall down…meanwhile I keep dancing." With four chauffeurs at my disposal any time of day, breakfast in bed, and gifts, not to mention support, feeling sorry for myself doesn't seem appropriate.

* * *

Dr. Kan comes across as a low-key, soft spoken man with a shy smile. He is the main draw bringing me to Sibley Memorial Hospital, now part of Johns Hopkins—that and the convenience of my family's proximity. Word on the street is Dr. Kan is one of the top GYN surgeons in the country. Mauri heard it from a woman sitting next to her at a restaurant bar. The woman overheard her mention Dr. Kan's name and interrupted the conversation to say, "Dr. Kan saved my life." Another family friend went to Sloan Kettering and was told she had two weeks to live, but came to Dr. Kan and was cured.

Since I consider my cancer's development a mystery, generated from my mind, I know I will be an anomaly to Dr. Kan. When I first admit my theory that my obsession and anxiety over the abortion targeted my ovaries and triggered cancer, a chorus rings out, "You're not that powerful."

"Oh, come on, the coincidence between my mental illness starting from my ovaries and my cancer staring from my ovaries doesn't seem the least bit ironic to you?"

"This is not your fault. You cannot give yourself cancer," Dr. Kan says flatly.

Damn, I guess if I can't give myself cancer I can't talk myself out of it either. What a juxtaposition. Cancer is going to help me overcome my feelings of loss, but I won't be alive to enjoy my liberation.

* * *

Todd is at corporate headquarters making sure life there does not become unhinged. Underneath my wish for him to show me he cares by unraveling, is the respect and gratitude I have for him maintaining calm. Todd will stay in the background as long as the four very strong women in my life remain in the front row. It works for all of us; it's a partnership Todd and I have agreed to.

My cancer diagnosis is like a hurricane. It is approaching New York as Todd prepares to pick Noah up from school. Meanwhile, I stand over the drawer that has been cleared out for me at Karyn's house. "What did I bring, what didn't I bring?" Clearly I wasn't anticipating staying very long. Not to worry, there is nothing my sisters won't lend me. My wardrobe doesn't surprise them; living in the Hudson Valley has humbled me. My toiletry bag doesn't take up much space on the bathroom vanity, since I only brought moisturizer. As I don't wear makeup, Mauri covertly applies base and eyeliner onto my blank face when I'm distracted. Magically a compact of blush will appear from her handbag. "Keep it," she says.

My internal alarm tells me it's three o'clock. Right now the doors to the middle school Noah attends are flying open and kids will disperse downwind like the white, puffy seeds of a dandelion parachuting into the streets and into their parents' cars. I don't know how many celebrate school dismissal the way I do, but today I pray Todd will fill my absence.

My secret to popularity with Noah might have something to do with the after-school treat. This expectation is exactly what annoys Todd about my parenting. According to him it is a hostage situation in the making. I'm already hostage by the mere fact that I am a mother who would move mountains for her child, so I buy him a cookie for a little display of his love in return.

46

Noah must be in Todd's car by now. How badly I want to call, but take in a sharp breath instead. Micromanaging this moment is out of the question. It is all up to Todd now; I wonder if he's scared. I'm not religious, but I pray. Please Todd, stop at the ice cream parlor so Noah can get a double scoop of killer chocolate and don't skimp on the sprinkles. Or take him to the bakery for a brownie and a bagel with cream cheese if he asks for both. Please do not put up boundaries today in which computer games will be prohibited and homework forced. Please do not argue, shun, use sarcasm, make him eat vegetables, or clean his room. Please do the following: hold him, tell him you love him, say he makes you proud, tell him how much you believe in him, and that life will be kind. Let him sleep in our bed with you tonight and every night should he want to while I am away.

* * *

It sickens me to do this, but I replay for my mother and sisters Dr. Laghari's message: gruesome words of advanced disease. At that same moment, I imagine Todd is telling Noah a softer version of the truth.

Tomorrow there will be a biopsy. We don't question the cost without insurance coverage in DC, and we don't ask questions about why it has to be done there at Johns Hopkins and why it is urgent. I could imagine my family thinking that this is no time to worry about money. I actually was afraid to bring up the concern for fear of seeming frugal.

6

HOW LONG?

September 20, 2017

The Voice Memos app is open on my cell phone recording the pre-show rambling of four women packed into the tiny exam room. The recording is not for me as much as it is for *The Isa Stories*. Walking through this ordeal as if it were fiction, doing it for the purpose of developing Isa has been an essential part of braiding our stories together. I'm only suffering on behalf of my character. When I go for a blood draw, it's Isa in the chair. After a procedure, I go back to the novel and replace inaccurate descriptions. Audio recording doctor's appointments helps with natural dialogue. When the book is complete I'll have learned all the lessons, the scenes will be authentic, but the experience will be over.

Dr. Kan has to squeeze through the door to enter. His amusement at my posse is humiliating. We find out that ten thousand dollars later, the results of the biopsy are inconclusive. He discusses, but does not answer the reason for the biopsy debacle. It is time to review my upcoming treatment plan and surgery. Before he continues, I pull out my questions—taken straight out of the ovarian cancer playbook.

"Laparoscopy or robotics?"

"We cut you open."

"How long can I expect to stay in the hospital?"

"Five to seven days."

"What is my recovery time?"

"Four weeks."

"Can there be a link to the fertility drugs I'd taken?"

"No evidence."

"Will you be removing the ovaries, uterus, cervix, fallopian tubes?"

"Yes and the omentum. There is cancer there too."

"How much cancer can you get?"

"In the abdomen? All of it." His eyes dodge mine. "But you started off with a lot of cancer, so much of it is already out of the barn. It's inoperable."

I hope to catch him off guard: "How long do I have to live?"

He gives me an impish smile. I assume he is being sensitive to my loved ones in the room. "I think a lot depends on how the disease unfolds. I think that certain people, if you're looking at the worst-case scenario, get treated with the chemo and it still progresses. It looks like you are looking for honest answers. It's an uphill battle to cure someone with stage four disease, as you know. It's hard. We're just going to have to leave it at that."

It is time for Dr. Kan to examine me so I politely tell the team to leave the room. As I lie on my back Dr. Kan fields more of my important questions including: "Can I receive Botox during chemotherapy?" and "Are you still sure this is cancer?"

"I see we're in the dark-humor phase," Dr. Kan replies, having seen this behavior before.

"Seriously, the biopsy posed a question if it is ovarian or cervical cancer."

"It's ovarian. Gilda Radner–type ovarian."

I put my pants back on knowing this is my last opportunity to rephrase my former question. As if I grab him by his shirt collar and pin him to the wall—in my mind—I ask, "How many years do you think I have? Worst-case scenario?"

"Two years." Then he walks out to make his next surgery, leaving his assistant to plan out the next year of my life.

* * *

Suddenly my humor around cancer isn't funny anymore. Half a marijuana edible is all it takes to jolt me into alarm. I haven't had my first round of chemotherapy yet and still have my hair, but today's appointment is proof enough that I have cancer.

I am in the kitchen when I hear Karyn answer the phone. Her voice goes up a register in excitement. I can tell she is getting some pretty good news about my situation, probably one of her friends who has a cousin who works at NIH and can get me in a trial if my first line of treatment doesn't work out. My brother in law calls out,

"Honey, enough with the oohs and ahhs." I hear her saying words like "wigs," "insurance," "chemo," and "long haul."

I stand here stoned and paranoid about having cancer and feel myself deflate—my honeymoon period has ended. Cancer is no longer mine, it is everyone else's.

I excuse myself from the kitchen, go up to the bedroom, and cry my eyes out.

Marijuana has brought on that sate of paranoia one might get from a police car flashing its lights and sounding the siren, before pulling you over. In this case, cancer is the cop car.

When I make an appearance downstairs to retrieve a glass of water, Karyn and Michael want to know how I'm enjoying my high. I have to confess it has suppressed my appetite and has made me a little anxious.

"If I didn't have cancer I probably would be in a really good mood," I tell them.

7

DEPRESSION CANCER

My real problem was mental illness, not cancer. Depression has come and gone my whole life.

It can't be trusted. At any moment I might be blindsided by a depressive episode that will put me in my therapists office a couple of times a week. It's a useless exercise, because my depression isn't controlled by talk therapy. Medication is usually the answer. Still I live in fear of these dark times.

Some of history's most talented writers have described the experience. J.K. Rowling once said in an interview with the UK Times that "Depression is the most unpleasant thing I have experienced...It is the absence of being able to envisage that you will ever be cheerful again. The absence of hope. That very deadened feeling, which is so different from feeling sad. Sad hurts but it's a healthy feeling. It is a necessary thing to feel. Depression is very different."

My calm, breezy attitude toward cancer isn't because I don't consider it serious or that I want to die, but because it is such a relief from obsessing over future decisions. It's an imperfect world, what can I say? If it were a game of *would you rather*: depression or cancer, I felt cancer would win. Anxiety had worn me down to threadbare. I was out of options and doubtful about my ability to move on. Every day my teeth clenched, my muscles tightened, I looked like a disoriented uptight turtle. Even when depression lost its hold on me, I knew it was lurking in a corner. Once that panic settles in your bones, you fear the onset of the next go-round. When I found out I had cancer, I thought, wow, I might never have to go there again.

My perception at age ten was that I would someday be the breadwinner of my chosen family. The image I had of independence was control. The only thing that could take control of me was my depression. My mom even referred to it as my "best friend," but then again, what best friend would suggest you jump off the subway platform?

I am a descendant of a long line of depressed, bipolar ancestors. There have been hills and valleys in my depression, but it is deeply rooted. When I was about thirteen years old my parents asked a psychiatrist friend to come to our house and speak with me. It was all so obviously calculated. He and I sat in the dining room. He asked me to, "Describe this glass," pointing to a glass of water in front of me. No shock that I said, "It's half empty." Suddenly, I was diagnosed with a chemical imbalance.

As a high-functioning person with depression, I have

always socialized, had boyfriends, and succeeded at work in a competitive field. When I met Todd he disputed that depression was real and bet he could replace my therapist with simple, carefree fun that required very little to no introspection. The truth is my therapist was useless, I would sit there in silence for 80 percent of the sessions, and so I was ready to stop going twice a week. Todd was so cute; his looks alone could distract me from brooding. I began to think of my years with him as remission.

One morning, a few months before my cancer diagnosis, I came down the stairs with tears in my eyes and an apology for Todd. I told him I had dreamed there was a growing crack in a paved road, too wide to jump and quite deep. The edges were jagged, making Z formations in the concrete. I spoke to my phantom dream companion, "See that fracture? That is my life."

Once I relayed this dream to Todd he offered counseling, not his own, but from a therapist. He loves me. He is my best friend, but no matter how codependent we are, he cannot share my depression. The crack may cross at our intersection, but that will be it.

The truth is that on a daily basis, the pain of depression is more debilitating than cancer, because I have had no symptoms of the latter. In this way I have to consider cancer a gift, assuming we coexist together for many years.

People suffer globally, from oppression, poverty, malnutrition, and brutality. I have a therapist, antidepressants, healthy foods, and a computer to document them all. I'll never know what true suffering is, or so you would think. With all the social and natural disasters in our world mental illness seems like a privilege. I assure you it is not. Cancer is and will remain a cousin of my mental illness, sharing a host, but separated by degrees. It is extremely unfortunate I have had to endure both. I have no control over either, but never, no matter how depressed or anxious I could ever get, would I intentionally or wishfully leave my child, my husband, my parents, or my sisters Mauri, Karyn, or Jill.

Each day I amaze myself. I am more aware, stronger, healthier, and happier knowing I have cancer. Contradictory to my condition I am thriving. Cancer and I are an oxymoron. This is how awakening happens, at least for me. Cancer's intention was to wake me up. Since I believe my emotional state manifested disease, my emotional state can eliminate it.

8

THE WIG

September 21, 2017

It is the first inning and my team is pumped with adrenaline, optimistic yet nervous adrenaline. I have just met with Dr. Kan, who will gut my insides and take out all my female organs. After a traumatic event like this, women have a predilection to shop. It can be self-soothing or a basic act of repression. There is some initial excitement about shopping for a wig, like we need a costume for *The Rocky Horror Picture Show* or the revival of *Hair*.

It has been a week, cancer and me. My sisters are anticipating cancer's sequence of events, therefore the wig. This outing is scarier than the impending surgery, because having a wig will make it all real.

Full of trepidation and a full head of long brown hair, I follow my mom and sisters into the wig shop like a duckling. I wish Todd were here to help. He is always honest. He never thinks it is necessary to lie, "When will it be useful?" How many times have I come home from a shopping spree only to hear him say, "I see you were shopping with your sisters again." I replay the whole trip in my mind and wonder at what point I thought the outfits looked good. I'm sure the committee who are now my "team" had something to do with it.

I want to dress like my grown-up sisters, neatly kept women, comfortably dressed for yoga, a cocktail party, or the theater. There are pictures of me as a two-year-old crawling toward them, a diaper sticking out of my Danskin leotard, my hair up in a ponytail, creating a fountain of tangled strands falling in my eyes and breakfast still plastered to my face. I have never successfully pushed past my comfort-zone of blue jeans, T-shirts, sneakers, or boots. One of the reasons I ended up in production is because of the casual dress code. All I needed was a fantastic buckle to make a statement.

This is just to say, when I sit down in the wig barber's chair looking like my two-year-old-self refusing to wear underwear because it is itchy, all eyes on me turn to utter dread and sympathy. The stylist, if you call her that, welcomes us with an arrogant, distracted smile. Frightened by my own reflection in the mirror, I look away. A brown-haired woman with a face of Styrofoam comes at me.

"It's real hair," the stylist boasts, "from Russia."

"Don't you have anything else?"

"Not real hair. Plus, this is the only one I have in your color."

The woman adjusts it forward and backward, and then rotates it. She steps away and extends her arms toward me as in ta-da!

My mom, "It could be your hair."

"It makes me look like a Hasidic woman."

"It's too thick. It needs to be thinned out," Karyn assures me.

Jill looks ashen and incredulous by the whole experience of being in a wig shop because I have cancer. I'm with her.

The stylist whips out a pair of thinning scissors like a gunslinger and starts cutting away. I own it now, I think, even though I haven't given her my credit card. The moment I see approved on her payment device, I feel a pit in my stomach. I'm not even going to reveal how much I paid: too much. My sister assures me it would cost twice that in Brooklyn.

9

SHOULD I FIGHT?

September 22, 2017

It wasn't exactly supposed to be a fun fall getaway in our nation's capital, but I was dead set on putting a positive spin on it. Todd, Noah, and Tom were coming to see me a week after I'd left home. Tom has only seen New Paltz since his arrival in America three weeks ago, so I arranged a tour of Washington, DC and sent Noah and Tom to shop top name brands at the galleria while Todd and I went to meet my new oncologist.

During the one week I have been in DC, I have met my surgeon, had a biopsy, bought a wig, and an iPhone for Noah. I did what?

"Todd, I bought an iPhone for Noah. Actually Mauri bought it, but it was my idea."

"I thought we weren't getting him one until high school?"

"I know, I know, but circumstances have changed. If I'm going to be away from him we need to communicate. He'll be able to FaceTime me."

"So you had to get him a phone? He couldn't use mine?"

"I want him to be able to call me whenever he wants. And I thought—I want to give him something to be excited about. A consolation prize. His mother has cancer. By the way, I missed you."

The next day, Karyn, Todd, and I squeeze into the exam room and wait for what I imagine to be the Wizard of Oz. He turns out to be a tall, gray-haired man in a white lab coat named Dr. Kohler. He squints at me and asks how I will pay for this. This? The consultation or everything, I wonder? It's as if he suspects me to dine and dash. I search through my bag and retrieve the coupon inserts I found at the information desk: coupons for the soup-and-sandwich combo at Au Bon Pain down the hall, not chemotherapy.

I tell you this only because it is chronologically important, albeit boring. I still have New York insurance that does not cover treatment at Johns Hopkins. To obtain Maryland insurance, I have to prove I live in Maryland by having a local address and a driver's license. Change a few credit cards to my new address, show a lease, and voilà, I become a ghost in my husband and child's life on paper.

The new insurance won't take effect for three months, which gives me a reprieve from being a castaway. The doctor's reluctance to see me without proof of payment strikes me as strange though: is his true concern that I will lower his patient-survival rate?

The only time the doctor meets my eyes is when I probe again about my time frame. "Chance," is all he offers. Not a "Good chance," or "You have a chance." There is no A in front of the chance at all, just "chance" and again that phrase, "It is very advanced." Whatever color was in Todd's face has disappeared. Karyn looks like a hurricane is coming and we've got to get out fast. But, wait, I haven't made the jokes forming in my head over the last ten minutes.

Dr. Kohler does understand one thing: being away from my family in New York is going to take an emotional toll and it (meaning everything) would be impossible to afford without health insurance. New York insurance will cover the first three chemotherapy infusions thirty minutes from home with Dr. Laghari, the oncologist who first spoke the words, "You have stage four ovarian cancer." When the Maryland insurance becomes active in December, I will be back at Johns Hopkins for the main event. I think of this three-month interim as halftime.

* * *

Leaving the hospital, I have never seen three people split ways so quickly. Karyn goes off to do some "errand" and Todd drives me to meet Noah, Tom, and my mother in Georgetown. We are both living a nightmare, but our dreamscapes couldn't be further apart. Breaking the silence, I ask, "Todd, what do you think you would do?"

"If I were in your shoes? I don't know if I'd choose to fight."

"So you don't think I should go through all the chemotherapy, everything it's going to take?"

"It's a personal choice. I support your wishes, whatever you want to do."

"So you don't think I should fight?"

"It's a rational decision."

My family would throw him over a cliff if they heard this conversation, but I am very protective of Todd.

Was I on a fishing expedition? I know Todd to only speak the truth. I am constantly weighing his truth against mine. He tells me not to buy whole wheat tortillas because they break apart. I buy them because they are whole wheat and then make my breakfast burrito. Sure enough it falls apart. I curse, "Why are you always right?!"

My husband is telling me he doesn't have an opinion one way or another regarding my will to live. Neither of us romanticizes old age and neither of us wants heroics to keep us alive if there is nothing to live for. Todd's father, who is now ninety-six, is still active and social, but he complains and has bouts of sadness. I asked Todd a few years back, "How can we protect ourselves from feeling that way?"

"I'm not worried about being ninety-two," he said flatly.

But I am fifty and my body still functions. I still have a 17 percent chance of surviving. What scares me most, however, is Todd is saying he wouldn't fight. Doesn't he know we need him? Suddenly, I am grateful it is me with cancer.

The car rolls to a red light at the intersection of Wisconsin Avenue and M Street. I jump out into oncoming traffic from three sides. I don't look back. I put on my headphones and find the perfect song for this occasion in my iTunes playlist. "Say Something" by A Great Big World. It bleeds into my ears and prompts a rain of tears.

Say something, I'm giving up on you
I'm sorry that I couldn't get to you
Anywhere, I would've followed you
Say something, I'm giving up on you
And I will swallow my pride
You're the one that I love
And I'm saying goodbye...

I am on my way to meet Noah at the Apple store; he is with my mom and Tom buying accessories for his new iPhone. Outside the store I wipe my face and hope Noah won't notice. There is no need to worry. The Apple Store is his paradise and the iPhone his sole preoccupation for the moment. He is the only one flying high today.

* * *

By nightfall, Todd returns after having a few. After he left me in Georgetown, I bet he stopped at the first shopping plaza with a bar. In his desperation even an Applebee's would do. Now I am sitting in Karyn's kitchen drinking a sixteen-ounce plastic party cup full of Tito's vodka. "Where'd you come from? I figured you'd find a bar after you left me. Did it have a good happy hour?" Todd dismisses me on his way through the kitchen. I'm bitter. Bitter that Todd didn't come after me, bitter that he went to a bar—without me, bitter that he is angry at me, bitter that I am holding a red plastic cup full of vodka because Todd drove me to it, and bitter that the one thing Kohler did answer today to, "Can I drink?" was "No." Well, Dr. Kohler isn't here to stop me.

My rage is bubbling. As Todd exits the kitchen I spit out, "How dare you be mad at me?"

Todd texts Karyn later that night:

> *I did a really dumb thing... After leaving the meeting with Beth's Dr at Sibley hospital, I stupidly offered up that if I were in her shoes I didn't know if I'd choose to fight or give up. DUMB! She naturally asked that if she chose not to fight, would I support that, and I said yes. I told her that it's a very personal choice and that I would support whichever decision she made. Well, this is one of those situations where it's not ok to go there. I should have known that sharing my view would get me in trouble. We were on our way to Georgetown and after hearing this Beth asked that I let her out of the car. I drove a few blocks and did. All I was able to say was that I didn't want to lose her, but I think by that point, my words rang hollow. What a fucking jerk I am. She asked me if I liked living and the best I could muster was "yes—on most days." Not a very smart way to counsel your wife who has cancer—dumb!!!!!*

Karyn's text back to Todd:

> *How dare you make Beth think she has choices at this moment? She needs to know you want her to do everything she can to beat this. She needs to know you love her enough not to let her make a choice not to fight. None of us knows what to say but that was the wrong thing. She seems so strong but she*

really needs you. I also know that you're a very rational thinker and you want Beth to feel she has control over her life. It's just not the time for that. It's time for all-out passion and understanding. I asked Beth to tell you what she needs but she is just so tired and scared and doesn't want to put you on the defensive. She really needs you and I know you need her too and that you must be exhausted and scared. But you show her how much you love her and want her to get well. That is my sister and I will do everything I can to protect her, you got it? Now is the time to show up and show her outward direct expression of love.

Todd was asleep by the time I came to bed, or faking it. I climbed in, my back facing his, and we waited for the sun. And it came. The sun, our apologies, our better behavior, and plans for a tour of DC on an amphibious Duck boat used in WWII.

That night we made up over a generous pour of straight tequila. I told him he could be unemotional and laissez-faire with the rest of the world as long as he wasn't that way with me. He put down his guard and I believed him when he told me not to give up.

10

LETTING GO

September 25, 2017

I know what I have to do. It is time to let go of a life not my own. Is this what cancer has to teach me? Is it so wrong to think it's arrived for a reason? Cancer parroted the voices, "Another child just wasn't meant to be." Now there is nothing to contemplate—not birth, adoption, not foster care. Is cancer my final punishment? Have I existed in prison for years and now been given the death penalty? The paralysis of my inner turmoil essentially is, as Todd has always warned against, a self-fulfilling prophecy.

Every three months for the past two years, Cornell's Center for Reproductive Medicine sends a bill for two hundred and fifty dollars. That is how much it costs to store my two frozen embryos. I let the bills accumulate and hide them under a stack of papers. It's not that I don't have the funds to pay every three months, it's that I don't have the resolution. I figured if I ignored the bills I wouldn't have to make a decision to let go of the embryos. It's my fine for the abortion.

Nothing changed when I started receiving notices from a debt collector on behalf of Cornell. I let them accumulate until I owed a sizable amount. Then I would pay it off and let the cycle start over again. This game fit the pattern of all my harebrained behaviors in the effort to torture myself: more debt, more heartache, more denial and magical thinking.

Just before my diagnosis, I got a phone call from what the caller ID identified as Cornell. Strangely, I was motivated to answer.

"Hello," the cool jazz voice on the other end intoned. "Is this Beth Cramer?"

"Yes."

"Ms. Cramer, I'm from the billing department at—"

I cut him off. "I know what this is about. I feel so sorry for you. I can't imagine having to call up vulnerable women all day, women who are emotionally torn about what to do with their embryos, but won't let go. Do you know how many women don't plan on using them? They don't. You have all of these embryos in your labs. There is no practical reason to keep them, but women keep paying the eighty-four a month ad infinitum hoping that the moment will crystalize and they'll find themselves filling out the disposition, checking the option box to terminate the storage, and stamp the envelope."

"Ma'am, would you like to make a payment over the phone now?" he asks.

"No, I'll take care of it later." I hang up.

The fact that the billing department makes calls to patients owing money for a variety of procedures, from gallbladder surgery to mole removal, never occurred to me.

The day before my first chemotherapy treatment, I settle my bill with Cornell and send in my consent to discard the frozen embryos. Would it really give me closure?

11

SOUL SCHOOL

September 26–September 28, 2017

I will never know the words Todd used to tell Noah I have cancer, but I know it took place during dinner at Mexican Kitchen over Noah's pork and pineapple tacos and Todd's fully loaded burrito. Months later I suggested to Noah we go to that same restaurant. "I'll never go back there. That's where I found out you have cancer," he said.

Recently I asked Todd, "Do you remember telling Noah I had cancer at Mexican Kitchen?"

"I didn't tell him."

"Yes, you did. I was in Maryland, remember?"

"No."

"You told him at Mexican Kitchen."

"I don't remember that."

"You don't remember being at Mexican Kitchen?"

"I don't remember telling him."

How could he forget? Conversely, why would he remember? This was traumatic enough for a bottlenose dolphin to block out.

* * *

Stepping back in time when Noah was a kindergartener at a Waldorf school, learning to bake bread, knit, and learn mythology, public school children were learning to read, write, and do some basic math. We were covered in fairy dust by all the Waldorf magic. There were Lantern Walks to welcome the winter solstice and May Day with an actual pole and daisy crowns even the eighth graders wore.

By third grade Noah's reading skills were just starting to emerge. In sixth grade, he told me Waldorf only teaches about gnomes and fairies and if you don't intend on growing up to be a craftsman the school is a total waste of time. What Todd and I had gambled on was not the academics alone, but the values that would nurture our whole child. The school considers the uniqueness of each individual and allows him or her to develop at their own pace. It is a complex and subtle philosophy, esoteric even, which leaves a parent completely in the dark about its effect because there is no objective measurement of success. So when our disappointment in Waldorf's methods reached a boiling point, we transferred Noah to the public middle school. He was in sixth grade. Now we were straddling both worlds, trying to hold onto the values of low technology and the new pressures of a mainstream society. When he left the Waldorf school, Noah didn't have a phone, computer, no email, no social media. Public middle school was academically successful for Noah, though his social life was a mystery to me. He began to separate from his core group of friends, essentially his brothers and sisters since kindergarten, and I was not meeting any new ones.

Cut to September 5, 2017. Noah enters the middle school as an optimistic seventh grader. He arrives on September 15 as a sullen boy whose mother has cancer and was swept off to DC. I envision the school hallways as danger zones. The middle school has all the makings of a horror film, with labyrinths you cannot escape and figures lurking in the shadows wanting to draw others to the Dark Side. What if Noah fell through this trapdoor, how would I get him back?

The middle school guidance counselor calls to tell me Noah sought her out and told her his mother has cancer. Noah had never met this woman before; I don't know how he found her. He spent over an hour in her office. He told her I was everything to him and cried. She tells me Noah used her computer to pull up my website and showed her videos I've directed and edited.

"He is so proud of you," she says.

"I am incredibly proud of him for having the courage to bring this to you and take care of himself," I respond.

Of course it will be okay, I tell myself. Look how Noah advocates for himself. He is resourceful, unafraid to show vulnerability, and has great instincts. It is me that I don't trust. How could I be certain his six new subject teachers and the hundreds of peers would care? I wrote them all lengthy individual emails. None of them could vouch for his safety.

It was my mother's idea to send Noah back to the Waldorf school. My mother has had very little confidence in Waldorf's educational system from kindergarten on, judging their strange and unconventional ways. It was the butt of many jokes. However, in that moment when I was struggling with what to do, she realized the school's gifts. Her support justified all the time I have spent defending Noah's education to my entire family. Strangely and inexplicably I believed when Noah finished fifth grade that he would be back for seventh.

With very little lead-time, I put together what amounts to an escape plan. Todd may not believe this execution is necessary, but he does not challenge me. My speech about Noah needing a school to nourish his soul rather than feed him Common Core standards is impassioned. Furthermore, I proclaim Noah's Waldorf teacher can act as a spiritual guide. With just twelve students in his Waldorf class, his teacher can monitor Noah's moods as opposed to the six teachers in public school who have twenty-four students each period.

Before Noah has time to clean out his middle school locker, he is back at Waldorf sitting on his *cajón* in front of a blackboard that has a beautiful chalk drawing of the Buddha on it. The *cajón* is a substitute for classroom chairs. Picture a wooden box about seat height. When you strike the surface between your knees, it makes a wide range of drum sounds. That drum chair, and the drawing of Buddha that Noah will replicate with his own hand, gives me solace.

12

THE MEDIPORT

October 3, 2017

After returning to New York, the effects of our meeting with Dr. Kohler still casting its malaise, I make appointments for chemotherapy and a procedure almost all cancer patients must endure. Patients undergoing chemotherapy have a device implanted in their chest just beneath the skin. In my case, you can see the catheter running up my neck and what looks like a stack of quarters jutting out of my collarbone. This is what I called a Metaport for a long time, before I learned it is actually a Mediport. Without it, blood draws, transfusions, etc., would cause collapsed veins. One thing I know for certain is that I do not want to die with this thing in my body.

Karyn and her dog Buddy stay the next three months in New Paltz with us. She gets me through my first chemotherapy and vows not to leave until my hair falls out.

After my first chemotherapy, I get my Mediport installed. The hospital in Kingston, New York, which is covered by my insurance, is in an impoverished neighborhood. I ask Karyn to turn the car around. It's bad enough I get queasy when I see an H sign on the roadway; this dilapidated structure requires a tranquilizer.

Entering through the main entrance, I am on the verge of a panic attack. The prison ward of a hospital room gives me a bad feeling. This surgery scares me. The Mediport will be a tattoo that says CANCER on my chest.

My surgeon, Dr. Katz, is a beautiful thirtysomething with long brown hair, a goatee, and a gentle bedside manner. Prior to the operation, we had met in his office where I had asked if the procedure would leave a scar.

"Nothing compared to the scar you'll get from the debulking surgery." Nice response. As I walked out of his office he noticed the Frye boots I'd bought in Nashville. "Nice boots. I like your style." I hoped this would give me preferential treatment on the operating table.

Then it came to me. My boots would serve as a symbol of my tenacity. At least I'd walk through this unfortunate journey in style. I did the calculation, a dollar a day for three hundred and fifty-eight days and those boots would be paid for with challenges, discomfort, soul searching, and trauma.

* * *

Lying back on the hospital bed at HealthAlliance Hospital in Kingston, NY an hour before the procedure, personnel swarm around me turning on machines.

"Which side do you want the port placed?" a young male nurse asks.

"You're kidding? Didn't Dr. Katz tell you which side?" I look bug eyed in Karyn's direction.

"No. I guess it's whatever you are comfortable with."

"I'm a righty... I don't know. I guess just put it on the left side."

"And what vein should I use for the injection site?"

Oh come on, I'm hoping *Candid Camera* is going to pull back the curtains now. Ask me to spell my last name or tell you my date of birth, but for god's sake don't ask me to make medical decisions!

The young man putting in the IV drip looks like a teenager. I can see the manifestation of his first mustache. He is studying to be a doctor and adorable, but I am wary of his skills. I ask him several times if he wants to call in a senior nurse for help despite Karyn's reproachful looks my way. His hands shake the more anxious I become. She suggests I take another Ativan. I hear him take in an audible breath before poking me in the arm and then release a breath out. "See? The drip flows freely." He lifts up the tube so I can see his success.

Only later do I appreciate this young man's sweet demeanor. Following my procedure, still sedated, I see him restocking medical tape. I wave to him, slur an apology for my behavior, and tell him he will make an excellent doctor one day.

After the Mediport procedure, feeling depleted and noticeably unstable, a nurse takes one look at me, one look at my shoes, and says, "I like your boots, they're very stylish, but I suggest you wear flats."

*   *   *

Now, several months after the Mediport was inserted, I reconstruct its significance. It is a portal into my soul, a weakness I do not wish to reveal. I recognize it every time I see a nurse approach. Like a dog cowering from its owner, aware that she is about to have her ears cleaned, I tremble. It took me a while to understand the waves of sadness that come over me in these instances. Why do I fear the port, when other patients seem to prefer it as a method for infusion? Why do I feel invaded and vulnerable the moment it is tapped?

I started to notice others' ports placed on the right side. A simple search on Wikipedia says the port should be placed on the right side to prevent it being damaged by the seat belt when in the driver's seat. That seems trivial compared to what an acupuncturist told me when I complained about the port. "It's directly over your heart center. That's why you're feeling such strong emotions."

13

ADVICE

October 10, 2017

In a rare moment I call Todd into the room to hold me. I am afraid. For my first chemotherapy treatments in New York, Karyn is still part of our household and I am spending more time getting used to seeing my bedroom during daylight. Todd and Karyn urge me to contact Erica, a woman who is the poster child for cancer in our Hudson Valley area. She has fought her cancer publicly, with Facebook posts of her bucket list, a column in the local paper documenting her journey, and photographs of her living *la vida loca* while receiving chemotherapy and radiation. I like this woman. Her courage and gregarious nature makes for a great role model. But I am not ready to reach out to other cancer warriors or survivors. Erica does not know of my diagnosis.

I agree to talk to Erica, but have no strength to compose an email so Todd writes one for me:

Hi Erica,

I hope you're doing well and I hope you won't mind my contacting you.

I have some unfortunate news about my health: two weeks ago I was diagnosed with stage 4 ovarian cancer. My doctors have recommended chemo then surgery and then more chemo. The reason I'm reaching out to you is that I'm scared and I don't know what I should be doing to keep myself strong. I thought perhaps that you would share some of your journey and personal experience with me in the hope that I may learn from you how to fight this thing. You seemingly have faced your illness head-on and publicly, and I respect that. I hold you in high regard for your bravery. I am still keeping my diagnosis limited to a close circle of friends and hope you will also keep this confidential. If you're comfortable offering me some counsel I'd really appreciate anything you can give.

Thanks so much,
Beth

I touched send without editing and five seconds later I got a response.

Wow. Now, good? I can call you whenever now through late-pm.

We spoke that night and it was just as Todd and Karyn said it would be, really insightful. When I told them of the things I learned from Erica their jaws dropped. The education I got was not what they were anticipating:

Erica is losing her "fight." It has taken over her organs, brain, lungs, and liver. She is one big infection, or as she phrases it, "one hot mess. Treatments keep going like a train wreck." She was making end-of-life plans. She chose a natural burial plot. These things hadn't even crossed my mind yet. Todd and Karyn would have grabbed the phone from me if they knew what was being said on the other end. But I want the hard truth.

"We are all going to die. No one knows how, but we do. We are not going to get hit by a bus. Our bus is here. Death is in our driveway." At this time I am reading a book by Bernie Siegel, *Love, Medicine and Miracles* in which he makes the case for mind over matter. I tell Erica that Dr. Siegel, like everyone else I speak to, believes staying positive is the key to getting healthy. Erica shoots back, "Positivity does not cure stage four cancer." I love her for saying this. What a relief! "Cancer is not personal, it's just doing what it does."

Erica sees me as a comrade, her disciple. I am just two weeks in, but as she points out there's lots of intensive treatment to look forward to. "The less they say the more they are hiding the truth," she warns about doctors. "Legacy work, do it now!" What is that, I wonder? "Make legacy boxes with letters written to Todd and Noah with pictures." She reminds me I am stage 4 so I better get my hospice care in order. Now!

Erica is adamant that I do hospice paperwork. Apparently, if I die in my home without it, there will be an investigation against my family; they will become suspects in my death. She wants to make sure I have that orange hospice sign on my door.

Years back I directed a music video that Erica's kids acted in. Since she knows me as a visual person she insists that I look at my CT imaging. She believes I could decipher messages from the cancer that the doctors are not capable of. By applying my perspective of structure, composition, light, and movement she suggests I can edit my masses and nodes together to tell a different story.

As of late, I have been questioning myself as a visual artist, but I want to buy into this concept immediately. An hour later my ambivalence kicks in. Truth aside, I am not ready to see the disease up close. But Erica wants me to stage a sit-in and tell my doctors, "I'm not leaving until I get answers."

Here are some of the questions Erica suggests I ask about my condition:

1. What does chemo and/or surgery achieve when there is this much cancer?
2. What is the outcome for the average person with this prognosis?
3. Give me a time frame!
4. What life do I want with the time I have left?
5. Will I be bedridden with treatments?
6. How do people die of my disease?
7. What is my life expectancy? (This was question 3, but it was important enough to reiterate, I guess.)
8. Find six pictures of healthy ovaries and six at stages 1, 2, 3, and 4.

9. Time frame?! (Again.)
10. Farm out the questions that feel overwhelming. (Good advice, Erica!)
11. Talk to Todd about end of life choices, for example burial, cremation, gifts.

I reached out to Erica and asked for counsel; she did not give me unsolicited advice. All the website links to cancer cures, articles, obscure vitamins, boxes of sea cucumber, and books about diet are not helpful. I want to see the article that says, "Are you searching for a miracle cure to cancer? Don't take my advice."

14

THE NUTRITIONIST, HOMEOPATH, AND ONCOLOGIST

What do you get when you put a nutritionist, homeopath, acupuncturist, and an oncologist in a room together? A mess.

Prior to chemotherapy, my first stop is to a nutritionist. My mom comes with me, prepared to take notes. We sit in leather seats and face the nutritionist, whose appearance is more lawyer or Wall Street broker than dietician. Her mahogany desk, framed certificates, and leather furnishings look more formal than I'd expected. She hands me forms titled "Policies" that read like a legal document with references notated at the end. Her vibe is a far cry from any hippy dippy New Paltz practitioner I have seen. She wears heels and a smart suit. Her nails are manicured. She has a business degree and an assistant.

She starts with muscle testing to determine an optimum personal diet, my best and worst foods, deficiencies, and daily nutritional requirements. The procedure, called kinesiology, consists of me extending my arm out and maintaining some resistance. The nutritionist pushes on my arm and asks, for example, does my body tolerate dairy? If my arm stays in place, the answer is yes. If my arm collapses to my side the answer is no.

I think we are off to a good start. Her first question is about alcohol. I didn't expect this to be open to debate. To my surprise vodka and tequila are a yes, but wine a no. More hard liquor, good. I nod my head at my mom and say, "Take a note of that." No gluten. No surprise. Other items don't seem believable. Like why would I not tolerate spinach but be okay with every other leafy green? Regardless, I sit back as she prescribes me thirteen different supplements that will boost my immune system and hands me a bill for a thousand dollars, which Mom pays.

I don't raise my eyebrows at the nutritionist's protocol. Why not? Because I have limited time with this professional and I want to believe she is a sorcerer. It is only thirty minutes after leaving her office that it occurs to me: a diet packed with orange juice and vodka—while I am grateful—doesn't make a lot of sense. Does she know I have cancer?

The first thing I do before making my way back to Karyn's is pick up a gallon of fresh-squeezed orange juice and a bottle of Tito's vodka, because the label says "gluten free." Once my cocktail is made the organizing of supplements can begin. I collect an array of Magic Markers and construction paper before sitting down at Karyn's dining room table. It is going to be a long night.

I've thrown out a few carefully crafted spreadsheets. Taking vitamins with meals is easy, when waking up and going to sleep, okay, between meals maybe, but there are several pills that don't fit into any of those time slots. The color-coded system I created shows thirty pills a day, plus powders, laid out in seven colors.

The day after I devise the chart, also the day before my first chemotherapy treatment begins back in New York, I send the list of supplements to my oncologist. He immediately puts the brakes on. According to him, supplements contradict the effects of treatment. Chemotherapy, or the preferred simile Pac-Man, eats all your cells, quickly devouring evil and healthy ones. Supplements boost both. To get maximum benefit of the chemo you must surrender without aid. With disaster narrowly thwarted, I walk into my first chemotherapy relieved of my supplemental burden.

There are other burdens coming my way. My sister Mauri gets a tip from an acquaintance with brain cancer. He claims that sea cucumber stopped his cancer from spreading. She asks me if I would use it and could she send some. "What is it?" I ask. She doesn't know but, "Why not try it?" At this point I don't object to this logic so I give a halfhearted yes. The next day Federal Express delivers a large Styrofoam cooler with dry ice packed around a six-month supply of individually wrapped sea cucumber capsules. This looks serious, like this could be the only food supply left if the earth is contaminated.

* * *

Whatever Todd is cooking smells good. Tonight will be my first dose of sea cucumber and I will eat it as an appetizer and delicacy. The shipment contains about twenty sleeves with ten tubs of sea cucumber in each, similar to a single-serve coffee pod. When I pull the foil top back, a disturbing smell escapes. The contents look like a frozen slushy. One, two, three, I throw it back wishing it were a shot of tequila. The gelatinous mystery of what I imagine dead fish to taste like slides down my throat. To get the benefit of this marine creature related to the sea urchin living on the ocean floor, I need three capsules a day. It has been used in traditional Chinese medicine for hundreds of years; no surprise it hasn't made its way to American supermarkets.

"Do you think three capsules a day is enough?" I ask Mauri instead of complaining. She hears hesitation in my voice.

"Each pod cost one hundred dollars, so tell me if you're not going to use it."

Oh my god, she could have told me that up front. Now I don't know what's worse, the taste of guilt or sea cucumber. The first few weeks I do shots of sea cucumber three times a day. Mauri periodically asks how it's going and even as I dwindle down to two a day, I say, "Fantastic." Karyn and I consult with another gynecological oncologist at Johns Hopkins, one of the top researchers in the country. "Is there anything I can do that's integrative? A special diet?"

"The dietary stuff isn't rocket science. Eat a variety of fruits, vegetables, and protein sources. Not a good time to be a vegetarian. There's no magic bullet. Kale for breakfast, lunch, and dinner is just punitive as far as I'm concerned."

"What about sea cucumbers?"

"I was an oceanography major in college and sea cucumbers are pretty gross, but do it if you want to." She gives me permission to say thanks but no thanks next time I'm offered a curative property. "If it is too good to be true, it probably is."

Back in New York I see a holistic chiropractor. What is supposed to be an hour consult turns into four. He agrees that I shouldn't add supplements, but has a lot of advice about diet that should include raw liver. This is an awesome, generous man who truly cares about his patients, but raw liver? I want to say no, but I feel like a coward. We discuss the Gerson Therapy, a much-talked-about protocol in alternative treatments. According to Gerson, using supplements, a special diet that consists of raw juices, and six coffee enemas a day helps the body fight its own cancer. Coffee enemas I learn are colon cleanses using actual coffee injected via the anus. This is a new fun fact. Thank you, cancer.

The chiropractor also provides resources for oxygen therapy, hyperbaric chambers, and cold-water immersion. Now down to eighty-five pounds, it's possible swimming in glacial water could kill me before the cancer does.

* * *

As I sit in the reclining chair at Dr. Laghari's office getting my first chemotherapy infusion, I see a text message pop up on my screen. It's from an acquaintance that knows about my diagnosis. Is he wishing me well? No, he provides a link to a video featuring alternative health and natural cancer experts presenting important information about healing and preventing cancer through diet and other alternative therapies. And let's face it, chemotherapy toxicity may be worse than the cancer itself. "Food for thought," my friend adds. Perfect timing.

This makes me recall a recent conversation with a Waldorf mother who told me, "Today I made sauerkraut, toothpaste, and yogurt." Two of the three I know are probiotic- rich foods. All around me people swig kombucha, another fermented drink with health benefits, so popular it's sold in gas stations. Our town has such a genuine hippie air about it that I'm wary to discuss my western approach to cancer treatment.

Flat on my back, needles deeply inserted into various points on my body, I rejoice in the pleasure of acupuncture. Moxa—think of a smoldering cigar—is burned directly on my skin. More pleasure, a hurts-so-good effect. Before I leave, my acupuncturist reviews dietary recommendations. Opening my notebook, I flip past the nutritionist's diet, the chiropractor's diet, and my oncologist's diet and find a blank page for hers. She prohibits coffee, alcohol, spicy food, refined sugars and flour, milk, yogurt, cold foods including raw vegetables, and salad. Yes to warm soups and stews, lightly steamed vegetables, congee, and steamed leafy greens including spinach. She advises me to go easy on salt, red meat, and no liver.

* * *

A girl needs some variety and tales of a new miracle machine that has arrived in town has captured my interest. Its purpose is to stimulate tissue to ease pain and presumably fight cancer. I rush through some precursory research to make sure Ondamed (Pulsed Electromagnetic Field Therapy) won't contradict my chemo protocol. It didn't for rats, so I schedule the appointment regardless of my knowledge that rats only have a two-year life span.

Most of my scientific proof comes from NCBI: The National Center for Biotechnology Information. It's brainy. I feel like a med student doing research in the United States National Library of Medicine or working at NIH. It's like knowing a little French and trying to read *Les Miserables* in its native language. You've seen the movie and the play, you think you know the plot, but none of it makes sense. What I need is an app like "Interpreter" that can translate medical documents into layman's terms. But I like to work hard, and one day I may understand gene nomenclature and the three billion letter pairs in our DNA.

The Ondamed machine warms up to do its work. The practitioner plugs several codes into the machine. She does not have a medical background, but she has a manual for reference. While frequencies pulse to deep regions of my body we begin to talk. This woman, so gentle and down-to-earth, made me want to open up and tell her the story of how I got here, starting with the abortion and ending with a cancer diagnosis.

15

DEAR PARENTS

October 18, 2017

The playground will buzz with questions about Noah's return to Waldorf; some close friends will get the true account. It is time to come out publicly with my cancer. It would be irresponsible of me not to inform these parents.

Like a getaway driver on steroids, I draft a letter to the parents in Noah's class the night before my second chemotherapy session.

Dear friends,

I want to share some information about my health that you may have already heard from your children. A little over a month ago I was diagnosed with stage IV ovarian cancer. While it is aggressive, I appear healthy and must admit I've never felt more clarity. There are many interesting things to investigate, such as how come my mind finally shut up, and will an illness as serious as this teach me that I no longer need to fix things, and can I finally release my grip and get on with living?

One of the reasons Noah is back at school is so that the people who love him most in our community may hold him. I consider Aram and your children to be his biggest allies outside my immediate family. Besides Todd, Noah is fortunate to be cared for by three loving aunts, his grandmother, and five cousins, though they are not local. The decision to move Noah back was so obvious to me. This moment is a time to feed Noah's soul and nourish his mind with a deeper education. As Noah told me himself, "The middle school teachers are there to teach, Aram is there to enrich."

I will tell you that Noah did very well in sixth grade, handling the transitions, the homework, the testing, the social scene, and all the challenges very well. This is a great sign for what's to come.

One month into seventh grade the pressures were mounting and then the news of my health made the decision to return an easy one. It's been my greatest relief in the scheme of our circumstances. I thank all of you for that.

This year we also have an exchange student from France living with us who truly is Noah's brother. Tom is the loveliest fifteen-year-old boy I have ever met and his spirit is an incredible gift to us all. He is going to New Paltz High School and will be with us until June. His presence is a stroke of luck or perhaps something more?

I've been thinking about what your children must be contemplating about illness and the proximity of it to their lives. I don't want them to be afraid or have questions unanswered. This makes me want to be very transparent with you so you can address those concerns.

I cannot take for granted the built-in support we have cultivated over the last seven years. We have shared so much and while I wish to protect our children, being aware of illness is inevitable; I hope with it comes positive views about living and the importance of friendship.

I'm a bit torn because Todd and I are private people and request that you keep our news confidential for now. However, I don't want Noah to feel burdened by our choices. He is free to seek support from whomever he needs to and I know he feels safe around all of you. Noah is very brave, but scared. His ability to express his feelings makes me very proud.

There will be a time when most of my treatment will be at Johns Hopkins in DC. This will be difficult for Noah and me. We are so bound together and separation will be very sad. He will visit on weekends, but having his Mountain Laurel family occupying him will lessen the pain.

I like to think a higher being, while not preventing me from getting cancer, is putting specific things in place to make it a softer landing.

To sum up, please don't be afraid to ask me any questions. I hope any conversations you choose to have with your children about my illness bring calm and generate some laughter. I've found laughter to be very natural in my own inner dialogue; it helps a lot.

Thank you for the many years of friendship and teamwork that have allowed me this privilege to share. Thank you for the safe place we together have harvested and for your beautiful children who are so empathetic and loving toward Noah. I expect to have many healthy years to watch our children grow and do amazing things. They are individually so powerful and together they are magic.

One more thing… I am taking a traditional western protocol for my treatment with an integrative approach. There is an overwhelming amount of information out there and while I appreciate all the holistic factors that could be beneficial, it is often conflicting. For now I have a protocol I'm happy with that includes chemotherapy and surgery along with shots of sea cucumber, acupuncture, oils, and a variety of other energy work and tinctures.

Todd and I need nothing more than your smiles, hugs, a walk when possible, and maybe a beer.

With much appreciation, trust, and love,
Beth

16

HAIR

October 20, 2017

While losing my hair is horrible, no longer having to worry about tweezing and shaving seems like a small prize. After my first chemotherapy treatment my hair had not fallen out. My oncologist warned me not to get cocky. "It will," he said. I lasted longer than most, but almost three months later it fell out.

Taking a page out of the how-to-prepare-for-chemotherapy playbook, I decide to cut my hair short before it all falls out. My mother advises me not to. "If you don't like the new temporary look, then you'll have two disappointments in a matter of weeks." Still I go for a pixie cut, shorter than I've worn my hair in forty years. Todd loves it and he doesn't know how to lie. Friends who don't know

I have cancer are complimentary, even envious. With each response I tell myself to be gracious.

My mom and Mauri are coming to be with me for the third chemotherapy treatment and get to see the cut in person. The photos my mom and Mauri take with me have this weird intention of preservation, yet who will want to remember the "cancer year"?

* * *

It takes me two days to get accustomed to my short hair. On the third day it begins to fall out in earnest. Although my shower this morning resembled an apocalypse, I want to hold out one more day before shaving my head of its remaining threads. Noah will be home tomorrow from a camping trip and I want him to witness my head shaving as liberation, not loss.

It will be the last time my hair clogs the drain in our bathroom. It won't be my hair on the floor or god forbid in food. Think of the savings on shampoo and conditioner, not to mention the products and haircuts. There won't be bad hair days. As I am losing my hair, Todd doesn't say a thing. Does he feel sorry for me? Is he starting to connect the dots between health and deterioration? What about our social lives, how will that change?

My shower, like those I read about, is a cancer rite of passage. My moment comes when the warm water flows over my head, taking my hair with it. My hands press the glass wall clouded with steam and leave a streak as I slowly lower to the tile floor in grief. I want to feel this loss profoundly. I want to earn an Oscar. I want to yell out, "It's not fair!" If I stay in the shower for too long all my hair will be gone and I need to preserve it for the next ceremony, the shaving of the head.

* * *

My third chemo appointment is today. The nurse gives me my premeds through the port; I feel disgusted as usual. Dr. Laghari appears. "I like your haircut."

"A preemptive strike. I guess you were right. I am not as exceptional as I thought," I say.

"Yeah, that's unfortunately what will happen. It will grow back. Different, you know? It could be curly or red. Yeah, lots of people have that. But it looks good, you know? Your hair short." I know, I know, everyone likes it short, let's see how they like the monk look.

Noah is expected home an hour after I get done with chemo. My mom, Mauri, and I pick him up at school. People might think I need to rest, but I'm proving to be a healthy terminally ill cancer patient. We pull into the school lot as the cars unload kids and their camping gear. Noah almost doesn't recognize me.

* * *

Although I could have a family member shave my head in my bathroom, I chose to visit a stylist. She had done the haircut leading up to this and we were bonding around the whole experience. After picking up Noah we head straight over. We pull into the driveway and everyone unclips their seat belts. To Mom and Mauri I say, "I'm sorry, I only want Noah to go in with me. Do you mind staying in the car?" I cower, waiting for a reaction. This shearing is not a party.

The shop is a one-chair salon, therefore very private. My butt hits the barber's chair and I know this is going to be something terrifyingly special. Like jumping into ice-cold water. A moment of awkwardness passes. Looking in the mirror is too much, besides, what is there to see? I swivel the barber's chair around to face Noah.

The electric razor buzzes, she maneuvers it in the air like a judge waiting to hit the gavel. "Are you ready?" Noah gives me the nod to go ahead and accompanies it with a smile.

"I might cry, but I might not," I warn him. He doesn't look nervous, why should I?

"It's okay, Mom. It's going to be cool."

"This is a great opportunity. When else would I ever get to see my head bald? It hasn't been bald since I was a baby."

"It's so weird and cool at the same time," Noah agrees.

"I'm ready." The hair hits the floor. I feel the buzzer close to my scalp, but Noah keeps genuinely smiling. I know the stylist is being extra careful not to nick me.

"All done," she says. Slowly I turn to face the mirror.

"It actually looks strangely good, Mom. Really, I'm surprised." Noah walks over to me, rubs my cue ball with fascination and more smiles, and then asks to have our picture taken.

17

ENEMY FORCES

November 8, 2017

The IV bag hangs on the pole, the drip chamber opens, and the pre-meds trickle into my bloodstream. I am powerless for hours as volumes drip, drip, drip. It makes me cringe when a friend tells me to thank the chemotherapy, to imagine it as healing light. People call me a warrior or brave; I want them to see me sitting in this La-Z-Boy. There is nothing brave about showing up for chemotherapy.

Drowsiness first, lack of coordination will come next. It is starting to kick in. My words jumble and unconscious thoughts rise to the surface. This is the fun part. It lasts for all of two minutes.

My eyes shut and an illusion emerges. A miniature version of myself is sucked up through the IV then deposited into my bloodstream. En route to the tumor I dodge the cancer cells that have metastasized. I'll come back for them later. Mini me holds an assault rifle targeting the tumors. I tell the healthy cells to stand back so I can take fire.

The cancer cells and the healthy ones look identical, but the cancer ones move around like they have a cocaine addiction. Once I've got one in my sight I shoot and they dissipate like an exploding star. One, two, three. I get four at once. As I maneuver up from the abdomen, circumventing the liver and lungs on my way to the chest and neck, all without GPS, I suss out the cells. It's hard to identify which side of the war they are on. I just have to open fire, casualties unknown.

In six hours the war is over, but some of the causalities will die slowly while others make it to medevac and prepare to get out of the field quickly. The army will once again multiply. Exhausted, my back slides down the perineum wall. I put down my gun. The sweat lingers on my brow. Looking down, I see the blood on my clothes and rips in my shirt that must have happened when I tripped over organs. I'll be back in three weeks with another infusion of chemical warfare and hopefully enough will to subdue the enemy.

18

MARIJUANA LADY

"Bye, Marijuana Lady," Noah shouts at the woman biking away from our house. Moments ago this woman, "Marijuana Lady," and I were holed up in my home office discussing a cannabis protocol to help me through my illness. Now I am stoned and praying she does not hear Noah's catcalls. A nurse oncologist turned cannabis advocate, president of a Cannabis Nurses Association, and "Glinda the Good Witch" in my cancer fairy tale, she also happens to be my neighbor.

Since first diagnosed, I have had a revolving door of friends gift me with high-quality products in the form of vaporizers, dose pens, tinctures, edibles, and joints. My small apothecary is lined up on the coffee table for "Marijuana Lady" to examine. After forty-five minutes of background, she gets down to business. Like a craps dealer at Vegas she swipes bottles to the left, joints and vape pens to the right. Raised eyebrows and a grunt tell me which goods pass muster and which don't. With each cut I feel the pangs of money gambled away on a losing hand. I knew I shouldn't have bought that weed from the anonymous woman I met at the infusion center who passed me a bag of nameless joints. That guy in Kingston who sold me oil he labeled "house blend" did seem shifty.

Without my medical marijuana license this meeting is illegal. In the age of "cannabis cures cancer," I am caught up in the excitement. But while cannabis is known to stimulate the appetite when a person is nauseated, for me it is an appetite suppressant. One night after an infusion I ate a marijuana edible and later fainted in Karyn's arms. Paranoia always threatens to crash my party. I've convinced myself that I have cancer in name only. If I was under the influence, there's a good chance I might trip into the real world of cancer. In a vulnerable state, "stage 4 ovarian cancer," will echo in my mind.

"Marijuana Lady" dismisses the idea that cannabis can cure cancer, but she is certain it will add quality to my life.

She spends three hours educating me on the properties of cannabis. I learn that the flower of the cannabis plant, nicknamed marijuana, contains both CBD and THC. They are basically two of eighty ingredients that make up the plant. Once extracted, THC and CBD can be combined to produce different effects. CBD is not psychoactive; it is THC that is responsible for the euphoric, mind-altering effects of the cannabis plant. A greater ratio of CBD-to-THC means less of a high, whereas as the THC increases, one will feel more psychoactive effects. There is literally a periodic table of marijuana strains.

It comes time for Marijuana Lady to show me how to operate the vape pen. She takes an enormous hit and indicates that I mimic her. Within moments, the room starts spinning. My guest becomes a two-headed monster. I'm afraid to speak and my anxiety increases tenfold. Admitting this does not feel good surprises her. She unabashedly tells me of her immunity to the effects. How much research has she done, how much can she tolerate, I wonder? I am losing confidence in my ability to follow the protocol and I am losing confidence in "Marijuana Lady" as a mentor. Her credentials no longer seem valid, but I'm stoned and remind myself that I'll question anything. She eyes two joints labeled Blue Cheese. "A good one?" I ask. She warns me against using it, but has no problem taking the joints for herself. As she pockets my Blue Cheese and other unidentified oils, I wonder where they will end up. Later I find out that Blue Cheese, a scarce but treasured strain, helped her through menopause. Nice trick: get me stoned and steal my best shit.

She recommends I take a hit of pure CBD to counteract the psychoactive effects of the THC and sure enough, it works. This is an amazing piece of information. If you feel too high you can always neutralize it. My vision stabilizes just in time for Noah to return home. No sooner do I recuperate than the door to the office flies open. John Wayne, aka my thirteen-year-old son leans in. "It reeks of pot." How does he know?

If there is such a thing as too much honesty, I am guilty. When Noah probes me about anything, usually none of his business, I feel compelled to succumb. What follows is a version of the truth accompanied by an explanation that opens a portal to more questions and more leaks. Noah often astonishes me with his knowledge of events and things he acquires on his own, but Todd insinuates that I am the informant giving away classified information to our son, confusing him as my equal and confusing him overall.

Flashback to Noah finding a stash of green bud in my closet. This was after my diagnosis. Although I had a medicinal excuse, I panicked. My poorly judged, think-fast response outed my brother-in-law, his uncle, as my source. Noah's face morphed into Edvard Munch's *The Scream* while I ransacked my brain for explanations. Once again I acted like an underage teen caught breaking the rules. Todd was not at all surprised when I relayed the episode. He looked at me and shook his head, sign language for, "You created this situation. Too much information, Beth, TMI."

I stepped into Noah's rabbit hole. "Noah, first of all: why were you in my closet?"

"Were you hiding it?"

"It's not about that. That is my closet and you don't have a right to snoop through it."

"I wasn't snooping. I was looking at the camera equipment."

Damn it, that closet was the worst hiding place. I store all my equipment in there. The gear fascinates Noah. It's his toy chest.

"Well...I'm not using it. That's why it's there."

Waving the Tupperware of green bud in the air, Noah

huffs around the room in hot-faced judgment. In his mind weed is an offense equal to cocaine or heroin. Calming Noah was no easy feat. He was busy linking any unusual past behavior with my "habit." He was angry that I had not confided in him about my usage.

Noah has a moral compass that puts anybody intoxicated, nicotine-addicted, or drug-addled south of his border. If he catches me having a glass of wine or enjoying a bit of chocolate he lectures, "You're not taking care of yourself, Mom! You have cancer. You shouldn't be drinking!" True to form, I always feel guilty and concede to his argument, which proves my weakness, allowing him to call me out the next time for what he regards as cheating.

Over the last several months, Noah has gone soft on marijuana. He began researching its chemical compounds and healing properties to understand how it might help me. I am proud of him for his ingenuity and possible future in the growing cannabis industry. He tells me while it's too soon for him to experiment, he may use it to relax in a few years or if I die he might just start smoking it incessantly to numb his pain. In a series of fast-approaching curveballs I get from Noah, I was not prepared for this one.

Whenever I get angry I hear my doctor's voice telling me it's important not to get agitated. Parenting a teenager and staying calm is an oxymoron. My option to ignore my kid's behavior or take a very long vacation doesn't seem realistic. Working with Noah on his homework, my impatience hit number ten on the Richter scale. All I could do was rub my hand back and forth over my smooth head, a comforting habit I picked up once I went bald.

"Mom, you have two veins popping out of your fore-head. Seriously, you should see it. Go look in the mirror. Am I making you that stressed?" Noah asked.

"Yes, but I love you."

"Well, why don't you go smoke some pot?"

19

PARENTING MY DOG

The day I find myself in the Tractor Supply store looking for mulch, I come across a litter of puppies at the end of aisle four. Though I did see the adoption event posted in the paper a week before, the thirty miles I drove for mulch had nothing to do with the puppies.

I left the store with a newly purchased crate and one six-week-old brindle mixed breed that looks like a Bengali tiger and no mulch. I drive home with a puerile smile across my face, proud of my fortitude.

A day after bringing Artemis home, I caught Todd speaking to him in that high-pitched voice reserved for pets and babies: "Hi, what's your name?" and "Who's a good boy? Who's a good boy?" Though he said he didn't want a dog, in a week he was posting cute puppy pictures on Facebook. He was the one that decided Artemis was the reincarnation of our much-loved Labrador who had passed two years before.

* * *

Just a year later, Artemis takes up the whole side of our mattress. If I wake in the middle of the night to go to the bathroom, I'm careful not to wake the dog. If the dog is awake and Todd asleep, I might be careless and drop a book on the wood floor. Artemis is maturing and has made the jump from our bed to Noah's, unless Noah is at a sleepover. Noah is a proud and loving brother, but I am still the alpha.

Artemis has also grown independent. Like most teenagers he's taken to wandering. At first it was just across High Pasture Road, which borders our property. Sometimes I'd get a call from a neighbor a quarter mile up the street informing me that Artemis was going to hang out for a while and was that okay. I'd find him with a young family in the midst of a birthday barbecue, Artemis comfortably sitting under the grill waiting for bits. The kids all call him by name and he ignores me as I arrive. I adore Artemis for his ability to fit in, but feel wounded that he seems to prefer their company.

Dog wandering was always acceptable when I was growing up. We would go to school and our dogs wandered the neighborhood, but came home for dinner and to sleep. Fear that Artemis could get into an accident, along with the judgment I faced from strangers, pressured me to create boundaries.

We got an invisible fence to save his life, I told myself. But I felt guilt for limiting him, as if I were holding him back from adventure. I knew I'd be robbing my neighbors, who are retired and value his companionship. He once lazed beside them as they weeded in their gardens. He relieved their empty nest syndrome.

Lately Artemis shies away from me. I am consumed with confusion and doubt over our relationship. Did he become wary of me when my hair fell out? Aren't dogs supposed to have a sixth sense when it comes to compassion and understanding? I was counting on him.

When I go to Johns Hopkins for weeks at a time, Todd is left to take care of Artemis. Everyone feels my absence and perhaps Artemis is rebelling. If I try to pet him, he flinches. If I sit down next to him he moves to the other side of the couch. Did I lose my familiar scent after chemotherapy? Does he know something I don't?

I'm considering therapy for the two of us. It's frustrating. All I want is for Artemis to lie next to me and cuddle. He seems to spend his whole day waiting for me to come home, but two minutes in he returns to his crate looking deflated by the realization that I'm not that great. He follows me around the house, but as soon as I go to pet him he moves away. I pat my mattress repeatedly and invite him up, but he just tilts his head and whines. Have I given a mixed signal somewhere down the line? I do talk too much. He is probably confused and does not know what I want. This would be better than shutting me out because I have cancer.

When he sleeps in Noah's bed, Artemis's head lays across Noah's chest. If my mom visits, Artemis lies right beside her without encouragement. He sidles up to everyone, come to think of it. Artemis is the sweetest dog according to anyone who has met him.

My loyal companion is supposed to be in tune with my feelings, he's supposed to comfort me. This is the agreement we make with our pets, isn't it?

20

COLOR WAR

There's nothing sexy about ovarian cancer. Have there been high-profile celebrities with ovarian cancer lately? Gilda Radner is the only one that comes to mind and she died in 1989. Mention breast cancer and it's a red carpet full of famous women. Granted, ovarian cancer is not as prevalent as breast cancer, in fact it's considered a rare cancer. I got curious about what I came to think of as Cinderella and the ugly, very grim stepsister with a grenade. I typed "ovarian cancer magazine articles" into my search engine and the first page listed *Britannica*, *MedicineNet*, *The Scientist*, and *Medical News Today*. I searched "breast cancer" and the results were *Vogue*, *Shape*, *Women's Health*, and *The New Yorker*. Now I don't like to complain about favoritism, but I am going to do an analysis of why breasts get all the publicity while ovaries remain so humble.

Breast cancer gets a color. Does ovarian cancer even have one? I looked it up, it does, and it is disappointing. Teal. Teal is my least favorite color—seriously. To make matters worse ovarian cancer's teal is so similar to prostate cancer's color that people can't tell the difference and they both share the same awareness month!

When I think of my sister's wedding back in 1989, my first thought is of the unfortunate bridesmaid dresses, the second is that it was a really beautiful affair. The dresses were constructed with a puffy sleeve reminiscent of Snow White, satin fabric covering my freshman fifteen, and a bustier that tightened against my upper midriff, forcing my breasts up while cutting off my air supply. I recall weights in the hem, which meant we couldn't run very fast, but the most offensive aspect to the dress was that it was teal. This is a color that belongs on no human body.

If I asked random people on the street what a teal ribbon stood for, I imagine few if any would have an answer. However, if they tried there would be a good chance of getting it right. Why? A teal awareness ribbon covers more than three dozen disorders.

- Agoraphobia
- Anaphylaxis
- Anxiety disorders
- Batten disease
- Child sexual abuse / assault
- Dissociative identity disorder
- Ectodermal dysplasias
- Food allergies

- Fragile X syndrome
- Gambling addiction
- Generalized anxiety disorder
- Gynecologic cancer
- Heterotaxy syndrome
- Interstitial cystitis
- Juvenile Scleroderma
- Military sexual assault
- MRSA
- Myasthenia gravis
- No Body Shaming
- Obsessive compulsive disorder
- Obsessive compulsive personality disorder
- Occipital neuralgia
- Ovarian cancer
- Panic disorder
- Polycystic kidney disease
- Polycystic ovarian syndrome
- Post-traumatic stress disorder (PTSD)
- Premature ovarian failure
- Premenstrual dysphoric disorder
- Progressive supranuclear palsy
- Rape
- Scleroderma
- Sexual assault
- Sexual assault on college campuses
- Sexual violence
- Social anxiety
- Stress disorders
- Systemic sclerosis
- Tourette syndrome

- Trigeminal neuralgia
- Women murdered by domestic violence

While I prefer not to be exploited for the benefit of companies making a profit off others' misfortune, it would be nice for ovarian cancer to have a share of advocacy, education, and visibility. With the publicity as it is now, at least I won't be bombarded with teal-colored products in every store window. Enough about teal—it's punitive, end of story.

21

MORNINGS LIKE THIS

On mornings like this I wake, my mouth parched. Sleep was elusive, my thoughts dull. Self-recrimination from my carelessness the night before lingers. Every night is suddenly the last supper. Wine flows once the bottle's opened. My self-control is like a leaf lifted by a strong wind. As a child I playfully try to catch it without real determination. Unconscious of time and self, I am free to run in unanticipated directions without any expectation of catching it.

There's no urgency to rise. Cancer is my birthday. Pillows propped, the extra weight of an afghan swaddling me, I will write today—after I reach for a book from my nightstand— *Radical Remission*, some light reading to sway my attention from cancer. Had I known it offered more integrative approaches to curing cancer with personal stories and protocols so diverse it's like ordering off a Chinese menu, I never would have picked it up. It really is a Chinese menu with a million herbal side dishes. Nothing's simple. Don't get me wrong, I'm a big believer that by integrating diet and spirituality there is a chance tumors could vanish without the use of chemotherapy and radiation, but conventional therapy is so much easier. Trusting alternative medicine is like using the navigation app Waze. You think it is going to save you time, but ends up getting you lost, turned around, and adds forty-five minutes to your arrival.

Still in bed reading *Radical Remission*, thoughts of tracking down the big five game animals in Africa and the difficulty of pursuing these enormous creatures on foot come to mind. Homeopathic approaches are abundant yet evasive. You should see my medicine chest. Abandoned vitamins, supplements, expired prescription drugs. If I dare to move one they will tumble like dominos.

My thoughts go back to alcohol. Once again I question its harm, pretending I don't definitively know. Hours spent searching medical journals for evidence that alcohol does not pose a risk has proved fruitless. Perhaps I should investigate French publications. Regardless, I scan the index of *Radical Remission*. Nothing, not one page dedicated to alcohol.

Guess what led me to delve into the ice cream last night? Alcohol. Even though it was vanilla bean, there was no excuse. Just last week my acupuncturist warned me dairy is the enemy. My team is losing, there are two strikes and it's the last inning. All night I imagined thousands of those little cancer cells bouncing off the walls of my stomach lining, high on cake and ice cream like manic children at a birthday party.

If my restrictive, organic diet did not protect me from disease, gluttony might. One article online said caffeinated coffee is harmful so I asked my nurse oncologist to confirm. According to her it's fine, as long as I don't drink eight cups. Cancer is the second leading cause of death in the world. There really should be one agreed-upon number of cups of coffee a cancer patient should drink in a day.

Twenty or more cases in *Radical Remission*, all survivors who mostly declined Western medicine, recount their secrets. No sweets, no meat, no dairy, no refined foods. That's a short chapter. All you have to do is follow your intuition, use herbs and supplements, release suppressed emotions, increase positive emotions, embrace social support, deepen your spiritual connection, and have a strong reason for living. Am I fully taking control of my health? I didn't know dying would be so much work.

For now, I'm putting my stock in emotional healing. Part of me strongly believes this is the end of the line; my final chance to let go and forgive myself for the abortion and the heartache my obsession caused those around me. More importantly, I need to change my perception of the idealized outcome I've hung onto for the past eight years. The termination of what would have been my second child broke me. Had that embryo developed and written a different story, there would be no regret. Our lives would have been storybook in this alternate universe. In this alternate universe I would not have cancer. If I could have stopped setting the table for four when it was the three of us sitting down to eat, I would not have cancer. The anxiety was too much.

Setting *Radical Remission* down on the bedside table next to two prescription bottles reminds me of my next task. Wellbutrin and Lexapro, my early morning birdsongs, a harmonic duet. I'll have green tea while I read the paper. A hard-boiled egg and an orange for breakfast. Has there been a study showing fruit and protein don't combine well? High-absorption curcumin capsules nag me when I open the cupboard, as does the vitamin D3, sea cucumber shots, and freshly pressed vegetable juices friends deliver. At the bakery where I do my writing I rarely order anything. Today on my way upstairs to claim my booth, I grab a cup of coffee with half-and-half and a glazed donut. Actually it was a honey grain roll with raisins, but it was not gluten-free.

I am on a writing tear thanks to cancer. There is so much material pouring in and all I had to do was change the proper nouns from Isa to Beth to make it happen. And then moments of doubt: when I go to the bathroom, when I go fetch a second cup of coffee, when I receive a text message, when I am putting on my shoes, walking the dog, I tense. Can you imagine if all I ever amount to is in this one book about death? And if I do live, then what will I write about?

My writing mentor, Abbey, asked me, "What's behind the humor?" I didn't know I was hiding anything. I really think some of this stuff is funny. What humor I could not find in depression comes pretty easily to me with cancer. It has been four months and real sorrow has not arrived. It's like feeling so sad you want to cry, but can't.

Now that I'm in a better mood, I can look back and find oddities in depression that might be funny. It was Noah who made me aware of something troubling about the way I process. "I remember you being depressed last year. You were making a ton of spinach, egg, and avocado sushi," he told me. Thinking back, I wondered why all those elaborate wraps tipped him off. For me this was a sign that I was taking care of myself. Instead I was avoiding work, the work I wanted to embrace but couldn't. Laying out the nori, placing the sauteed spinach on top of the avocado and scrambled egg, wetting the bamboo matt and rolling the ingredients, sharpening my knife and carefully cutting it into pieces, held some kind of sadness. Did Noah sense disillusionment in my preparations? Was my ennui on display all that time? He saw it, I'm sure of it, and all the times before that, he saw.

Noah holds a lot. Can he also see the cancer as a correlation to depression? What about the drinking? Tonight I won't drink. In fact I will not accept any invitation that might involve drinking. In a way I thank God for chemotherapy, it naturally forces a sober period. You can always tell I'm over the hump of its side effects when the fermented grapes pass my lips. Noah's scolding last night still rings in my ears.

"Mom, you're not taking care of yourself. Wine is bad, especially while having chemotherapy, and now you're having ice cream." Am I empowering him in a negative way if I plead guilty? And then what, when there is a next time? There will be a next time, I tell myself. It reminds me I'm living.

22

TEN REASONS

My therapist suggests I see someone new. She isn't firing me, she merely feels traditional psychotherapy is not working. Joy, the new therapist, is an energy healer. Hoping she is a wizard who will transform me without my participation sounds good to me. Before Joy begins I ask, "Do I have to believe in this for it to work?"

She tells me to shut my eyes. Her voice comes through in a melodic whisper: "Imagine a big puffy cumulus cloud above you the length of the table. Put each of your thoughts into the cloud, all your negative energies into it, and let the cloud carry them away." I panic. What if the clouds move on before I put everything in it? She must have read my mind, because along comes a small cloud just in case I find more to discard. It feels like trash pickup day and I do not want to be left with rotting garbage in my closet.

Joy begins to ramble in a language that sounds like something between Hebrew and pig Latin. I peek. Her eyes are closed. Joy welcomes my spirit guides. Mary, Gabriel, Peter. They are all so, so Christian, I think. I expected a Jewish lot, like Abraham, Anne Frank, maybe Elie Wiesel. With no knowledge or connection to Mother Mary, I am skeptical, but this is Joy's show and I can't change the characters mid performance. So, believing she and the spirit guides will work it out, I fall asleep.

After Joy releases me from my trance, she looks at me with what I take to be trepidation. "You have been out of your body for a very long time. I got you grounded for the moment." Then come the words no patient wants to hear from their therapist. "I have to tell you, I've never had a patient with so much blockage. You have to start speaking up for yourself."

"I don't have a lot to say; that doesn't mean I haven't been speaking up for myself," I say in defense.

"You have a lot of work to do in a short amount of time." We schedule our next session for the following week.

As I collect my coat she gives me an assignment. "I want you to write down ten reasons for living and bring it to our next session." I sit there, dumb. One of my spirit guides Mary, Gabriel, or Peter must have blabbed. This assignment is pointed. It is not going to be easy and she knows it.

Soon after being told of my cancer (I call this the honeymoon period), my vision was perfect, the clearest it had been since I was six. Walking my dog down Pine Road a tree caught my eye. I have passed that tree a hundred times, but this day it transformed into a splendid fairy tale tree. I looked up to check the sky. The sky was fully saturated with deep blue. It was glorious. I looked back to see my dog happily sniffing a tree. I smiled without feeling a bit of envy for his simplistic discoveries and time to acknowledge them. Spontaneously, I started skipping backward. It didn't matter that people walked toward me. I was—what do you call it—umm—I think—no, I know. I was happy. My face looks smoother when I look in the mirror. I don't want to drink, medicate, or smoke anything that will alter my crisp mind. It's as if I searched the world over, dying to find clarity, only to find imminent death was what it took.

On the way home I felt an eagerness to play the piano, something I haven't done in years. I sat down and composed a song as if it were 1985. This feeling was a small miracle, one I wanted to last. Maybe this time it would because clearly cancer was my emancipation. But after a couple of months I couldn't hold on to the intention. One night Todd asked me if I wanted meatloaf for diner, and I said yes. Oh my god: Joy, the therapist, was right! I don't speak my truth!

* * *

Ten reasons. Noah's name takes up every line. I have to try harder. What if someone actually sees this list? Family and friends take up lines two and three, but then in a moment of hope, I group them together. For days I rack my brain. There are so many things to consider, but I want them to be authentic. The therapist said I was out of my body. She was right. It made me think: isn't it crazy we even have a body? Look: I have hands, but this is way too broad to itemize. I have lists started in various notebooks and on the backs of receipts. On day three my list has: 1. Noah, 2. Todd, 3. Mom/sisters/Dad/friends, 4. travel, 5. glazed do-nuts—What? I can't remember the last time I had a donut, maybe 1985?

Todd has a catalog of reasons not to travel. I promise him I won't keep bringing it up, "but why don't you want to travel with me again?"

"It's not that I don't want to travel *with you*, it's that I don't like to travel. But while I'm not willing to go to Europe, I can give a wholehearted yes to making a trip to Dunkin' Donuts with you."

My writing mentor makes number six on the list with-out hesitation. When I met her my feelings of first love and possibility blossomed. She inspired self-confidence. Abigail Thomas, Abbey, is a writer I came to admire im-mediately after attending her writers' group and then reading one of her many memoirs, *Safekeeping*. During a bold moment I asked her to be my mentor and she agreed. My reason to write became twofold. I wanted to impress Abbey, create reasons to build our friendship, and com-plete a book. It was a beautiful start sitting next to her on her couch as she chain-smoked Marlboros, her three dogs jumping on and off the sofa while we conversed about my work and life. Abbey ended up having some health issues and family business that put our meetings on hold. I wonder, if everything I put on my list isn't permanent, should it be considered?

Just a day before my assignment is due my list is com-plete: 7. accomplishing something, 8. the possibility of en-lightenment, 9. the possibility of finding my passion, and 10. Noah.

Adding "the possibility" before reasons is definitely cheating, so they have to be scrapped. Then I remember skipping backward. It is possible to lower my expectations. Spontaneously skipping goes on the list. I walk into Joy's office and say: "Even if nine different reasons don't fill this list, I'm good with writing Noah ten times."

23

TRAVEL THE ILLUSION

December 1, 2017

My vision of enlightenment is to climb a high peak in Nepal, be welcomed by a monk, and walk along the colonnade, my hands clasped behind my back, eager to receive wisdom.

"You say that all the time."

"I do?" I ask my friend Alan as we walk our dogs. Alan is seventy-five, we walk and talk for an hour almost every day, barely taking in a breath. His musings and mine flow with each step. We are playing monks. One of the things I really admire about Alan is that he doesn't wear shoes, ever, not in the snow or on a rocky trail. So when I keep threatening to seek a shaman in a far-off land to teach me my truth, he says, "You are in it. You are walking it this very moment."

"I know...I know! Why can't I get that through my head?"

"I don't know. Why?"

"The path, for me, is just part of the game. There are rituals along the way that I have to pass before the moment of truth. I want to be at least partially prepared when the mystery of life is revealed to me."

Do I have a bucket list? Yes, now I do. The list rotates around travel. Anytime I hear of a new destination, I jot it down in my notes app: Budapest, Prague, Vienna, Croatia, Vancouver, Thailand, South Africa.

I was ecstatic and surprised when Todd gave me an issue of *Travel + Leisure* magazine as a birthday gift a few years ago. With anticipation, I flipped through the issue expecting airplane tickets marking a featured destination to drop out. I pictured a note saying, "Happy Birthday! We are celebrating in ..." But there were no airplane tickets or itineraries stuffed into the pages; the gift was the magazine itself and a subscription for the year.

* * *

Between chemotherapies, Karyn and I drive back to DC to meet a research oncologist. In the waiting room the coffee table overflows with magazines. The only subscription they have is to *Travel + Leisure* and it is a vast collection. My treatment schedule is so tight that travel is unrealistic. What If I don't live long enough to see these places? These magazines taunt me, I feel insulted, like seeing an invitation to a birthday party but knowing I am not invited. Begrudgingly, I finger through the pages. I may be imagining things, but the feature article is about Nepal, with a photograph of a monk and someone with my profile deep in meditation. All these travel magazines bring up questions about time, the idea of making plans, a bucket list. Waving the magazine in Karyn's direction, she catches my disapproval.

* * *

My family's concern for my weakened immune system fires up whenever I start to book public transportation. My mother tells me she will have a heart attack if I fly or take a train, as if I were Tod from *The Boy in the Plastic Bubble*. A picture of me snowboarding posted on Facebook three days after chemotherapy did not persuade her of my fortitude.

For Todd's birthday I propose a romantic getaway to Virgin Gorda: beach hopping, scuba diving, rum by the ocean, calypso at night.

"Too long of a flight," Todd decides.

"Montreal?"

"In December?"

Karyn is witness to some of our conversation and later confides in Todd that these trips aren't exactly about him.

* * *

It must have been the wine. I shouldn't have been drinking, at least not that second glass. I was high on the illusion of romance even with cancer, the illusion that I was not bald and my bikini wouldn't soon expose a scar mapping an eight-inch trek from pubic bone up my torso and beyond my belly button.

The mail truck doesn't deliver travel magazines to my home anymore and although the tabs to "World's Best Romantic Islands" and "Places to Visit in 2018" pop up on my browser, I avoid engaging in the dream; instead I'm beginning to have a profound experience through meditation.

Yesterday I was able to visualize myself in the lotus position on a large flat rock facing a cascading stream. Water rushes from a great block of ice hanging from a branch like Rapunzel's hair. Snow clings to rocks interspersed throughout the streambed. I sit in a glass box, the image of purity, protected from cold and air. My conscious mind wants to invite the fresh air to inhabit my lungs, but I cannot alter my initial vision. For a moment I wonder how I might paint the scene, but force my attention back to the creek.

Today's meditation went further. While I start in the glass box, the sides collapse and winter turns to spring then to summer. I am bathed in a shaft of light. Flat on my back, I lie in the middle of a stream while water flows around my curves. The droplets of water smooth my hair into silk. My mind wanders, but comes back to find me standing underneath a strong waterfall. The commanding rush is just a foot or two from my face, but I am not afraid of its power.

What happens next is truly an epiphany. I become the water itself. I am energy, an endless flow. Aware that I have no solid form, that I left my vessel, is a small miracle. I didn't turn to stone. I had the power to transform with just my mind.

24

SEX

A few weeks into my cancer journey I feel liberated from ambitious aspirations. It is comforting to accept the ordinary as profound. Finally the possibility of death sways me to live in the present. So when Todd drives me to my CT scan I remember to mention the tire pressure warning that appears whenever I start my car. My tires needed changing five thousand miles ago.

He asks me some rudimentary questions regarding the tires, which I feel is cruel because he knows I don't have the answers.

"I'm going to learn about my car. Maybe it's time for me to grow up," I tell him.

"Why bother?" he replies and we laugh.

At dinner one night, I ask him about the ingredients in his chicken marinade. I am concerned it might be Stubb's, which has so many preservatives.

He replies, "What, you worried about dying?"

This too makes me laugh. When's the last time we laughed at each other's jokes? I find this kind of teasing endearing. To me it means trust. When I first went bald, Todd announced that he woke that morning shocked to be sleeping next to his father-in-law. Apparently, without hair, I look like an eighty-five-year old Jewish man from Philadelphia. This last truth, though still humorous, brings up aspects of cancer that are difficult to face and difficult for partners to face.

Am I not still me, if not a better version? Will I lose my inhibitions? Be open to exploration? Who will see me the way I am ready to see myself, not someone who is dying, but someone who is truly living?

How can I expect my overnight change to transform my partner? It takes courage to change in view of those who think they know us best. It's easier to pretend there is nothing more to know. Todd and I share a bathroom, I watch him cut his toenails, and we know sex will often be predictable but tender. There's comfort in that—or is it an assumption our partner will reject something new? I fear humiliation.

Todd and I learned on our first date what music the other likes. Our tastes defined us. Would we be disappointed or feel insecure if our tastes changed? When I express new ways of thinking since we married, it's often met with disbelief. My tastes have changed. I continually have to remind him that people, women especially, evolve over time. We find this fun. Men: please keep up.

In my twenties, I was just getting to know my body as a woman. New lovers gave me my only practical education.

Now, I find myself fantasizing about reinvigorating my sex life with Todd. It comes to my attention that my timing is off. The physical attributes of cancer are a foreplay stopper.

25

FAITH

December 15, 2017

One day, I saw a listing in the local newspaper for a contemplative Shabbat morning service with Rabbi Rita Rosenthal. JUDAISM AND THE MYSTERIES OF LIFE, DEATH & THE WORLD BEYOND. Jackpot! This would make a great scene for *The Isa Stories*.

Stumbling across this notice is a miracle in itself. Surely God has something to tell me—I mean Isa. I am not an especially observant Jew, but perhaps there will be something to learn about faith. I'm not sure about Isa yet, but I'd really like to unlock the mystery behind my illness.

Upon entering the building, I see twenty-five folding chairs arranged in a circle and I tense. My image of anonymously slipping into a pew has vanished. People in their late seventies and eighties mingle in small groups. As I start backing out, a hunchbacked woman named Edna sweeps me into her orb and hands me a name tag. I write ISA in black marker and stick it to my chest.

A woman's voice sings nonsense syllables, "Ya did de da, did de da," the Hebrew version of yodeling or "la la la." I recognize this as the cue to take our seats. The rabbi, a woman wearing a yarmulke, prayer shawl, and Birkenstock sandals, welcomes us. "Shabbat Shalom," she says and without any preamble leads us in a prayer. I know some key words in Hebrew and sing the blessings. Even the ones I don't remember I can fake.

"I'd just like to go around the room, and if you feel inclined, say something you are grateful for," the rabbi offers.

Surveying the room for an escape route, my eyes dart around the circle of unfamiliar faces expecting to find looks of desperation, loneliness, and lack of hope. Why, because they're old? I'm the only one who looks like a deer caught in the headlights.

One woman begins: "I'm getting pleasure and I am grateful for so many warm and friendly people surrounding me."

A man with dry mouth goes next: "I'm happy my wife and I have this community. I've made many connections and feel very comfortable here."

His wife: "I'm thankful for walking in the mountains and looking at all the springtime flowers."

It's my turn. All eyes are on me. I think back to my ten reasons to live. I'm flooded with guilt. I'm just here to get a story, I want to tell them. My contemplation is taking too much time and the rabbi passes over me with a sympathetic nod. I am relieved when she begins her sermon.

"So Judaism and the mysteries of life, death, and the world beyond. I know: big. Way too big to get through in one morning service. But this is a series and the community is welcome to come to one or all of the sessions. So this morning I am here to address the question of all questions, the big conundrum. So you want to know the meaning of life?"

Yes, please, but I'd like my dressing on the side and just the lettuce.

"I think, 'How can I make my life more meaningful?' is the real question," Rabbi Rita offers.

Wait, what? That sounds like work. Death just let me off the hook. I don't want to find meaning. I want to live in the moment.

"Clearly nothing makes us look at life and its meaning more than death."

What did I just say?

"The great paradox of the Jewish brand is that life and death are deeply mysterious. Faith begins in mystery."

It occurs to me that what I have been lacking my entire life is faith: simple black-and-white, clear-cut faith, not debating where I am supposed to be or who I am supposed to be. Who will I be once I die? Jews have no answer to the afterlife, just more interpretation. Do I have time to invest in spirituality through Judaism? I love nothing more than a good midrash, but cancer quieted my mind and life just stopped being so ambiguous. Can't I just be baptized?

Announcements are made. There will be a senior luncheon on Tuesday, January 13. The rabbi looks directly at me. "Doesn't just have to be seniors."

Someone in the group reminds everyone to come to the Death Café at the retirement home. I have no idea what this is, but I like a latte. Plus, I'm still thinking of Isa. If nothing else it will make for a good scene.

26

MILESTONES

Leading up to my thirteenth birthday, I spent months preparing for my bat mitzvah: learning to chant my Torah portion in Hebrew, writing a speech, and planning the party. I remember the pride I felt after successfully pulling off this feat. It was not about God; it was about having a Jewish identity. If I meet another Jew who had a bar or bat mitzvah at thirteen I get a pretty good sense of what they felt like as a gawky, awkward teenager standing up in front of their friends and family. As an adult, I've started to resent the shotgun bar mitzvahs some kids have for the money and party alone.

I recently attended one of Noah's friend's bar mitzvah. It was far from lavish and everything about it was meaningful. When Eli and his mother stepped onto a makeshift bema (the service was held in a community center), the heat in my chest and my tears surprised me. Eli's mother radiated a mixture of pride and sadness. This is the bittersweet moment when a boy becomes a man in the eyes of God and his community, even if he hasn't gone through puberty. She is acknowledging her son's independence. It's like giving him a certificate of maturity. To me it represents a separation I am not ready for. This moment created conflicting emotional drama.

Why wasn't I pushing Noah to be bar mitzvahed? Will he not become a man if he skips this rite of passage? Am I afraid to accept Noah needing me less? How can I subject Noah to Hebrew school when regular school is hard enough? Noah won't know what he's missing if there is no bar mitzvah, but I wouldn't be doing my job if I didn't offer him the opportunity to experience it.

I keep telling myself it doesn't matter if he is thirteen or twenty when he gets bar mitzvahed, if at all, but that's a lie. I want to appeal to Noah by telling him what it would mean for me to see him bar mitzvahed without mentioning my illness. Isn't this as much a milestone for me as it is for him?

In the past our conversation about Judaism would go something like this:

"Hey Noah, would you consider going back to Hebrew school?"

Noah: "No. I hate God."

"Why would you say that?"

"How could a god allow all those people to die in the Holocaust? Why were the Jews always punished with floods and locusts? He's an asshole. I hate being Jewish."

I argue, "Noah, if you had been born sixty years earlier, you might feel differently. You are a Jew and would have been seen as a Jew and understood Judaism given the circumstances." Even I don't understand what I just said. My complex explanations always seem to miss the mark.

Hadn't I been the one to let Noah drop out of Hebrew school, to denounce Judaism and put the whole issue on the shelf? No one besides me is going to drive this boat. How many times have I overheard Noah tell his grandparents that, "In his family they don't eat processed food," or that "It's important to be kind to animals and regulate yourself when it comes to sweets and video games." Ha, proof that my morals have seeped in, regardless of Noah's indifference to these rules at home.

Recently, Eli, Noah's friend who was bar mitzvahed, spent the day with us. Still ever the boy, he recounted his gifts: the Legos he still enjoyed, the Nerf guns, and the money—a lot of money. This piqued Noah's interest, an angle I hadn't anticipated. The promise of cash may be enough to reel him in.

Before I could use money as a reason I had to go ahead and explain the importance of having a spiritual education. So stupid. The only way I convince myself of anything is to hash it out with my thirteen-year-old, a mistake anyone can see from a far distance. I really believe he deserves to understand. Time and again, this approach backfires.

One evening I entice Noah into a card game and approach the subject of a bar mitzvah. One round in:

"Noah, what do you think about having a bar mitzvah?"

"Maybe."

"Okay, that's better than 'no.' I'm curious"— I'm proud of myself for remembering the key words from *How to Talk So Kids Will Listen*—"what do you think about the idea?"

"How much money do you think I'll get?"

"I don't know. I guess it depends on how many people we invite."

"Eli got four thousand dollars."

"I can't promise that, but it will be way more than you have now."

"Will I have to put it all in my college fund?"

"Some of it."

"Like what, fifty percent?"

"You'll be able to spend a lot of it the way you want and the rest would be held in the bank."

"Like a hundred? I could keep a hundred?"

"Sure."

"Two hundred? Could I keep that?"

"Probably."

"Then three hundred. Let's say I could keep at least three hundred."

"Noah, you'll get money."

"Okay."

"You'll have to study, but we'll find you a rabbi that you like."

Did I not hear him say okay? Noah acquiesced only seconds ago, but now looks up at me with antipathy.

"I don't want to go to Hebrew school. It's a waste of my time."

"It's a spiritual education. It's important to consider things in life like morals and values."

"Fuck that."

"Noah!"

"I hate being Jewish. It's going to take up so much of my time."

"Being Jewish?"

"I'm out of here." He tosses his cards on the table and storms off.

"It will matter to you when you're older," I yell after him.

"Right. You always say that."

"Well, it means something to me."

Noah stops in the doorway, just feet from where the Xbox awaits. "Why, so you can be proud of me?" He lays "proud" out like it's a big insult.

"Yes. I'm proud of you no matter what, but I'd be proud of that accomplishment."

"You're wasting my time. Just talking about this is wasting my time."

"It's also important for your grandparents to be able to see you bar mitzvahed."

"Before they die?"

"Yes. It's a long-standing tradition and it's a milestone that would be nice for them to know you went through while they're alive." I really mean while I'm alive.

"I'm done playing. I'm going back to my Xbox."

"See?" I call after him, "You could use a spiritual education! Your relationship with your computer game is more important to you than your relationship with me."

Did I just talk my son out of a bar mitzvah?

27

LEGACY BOX

I woke this morning strong enough to hover over the stove for forty minutes making breakfast and lunch for Noah and Tom. Tom catches the school bus and but I drive Noah to school. Suddenly I am pulled down a black vortex of nothingness. Staggering to a bench, I land just in time to lose consciousness.

"Mom, Mom?" Noah pleads. "Hang on. Don't move." I sense him running out the kitchen door yelling, "Dad! Dad, come quick." I raise my head from between my legs to see Noah standing over me, his fear palpable. Todd moves into frame, for I am surely watching a movie and not my life.

"Mom, you had a seizure. That's it; I'm not going to school. You can never be left alone. You had a seizure!"

"I did not, Noah. I just felt dizzy. That's why I moved to the bench."

"Your eyes rolled back and you were shaking."

"I may have fainted."

"I know what a seizure looks like."

"Okay, okay," Todd referees. "Noah, Mom's going to rest. Let's take her to the couch." Todd takes hold of my arm. Noah's spots me as if I am doing a triple back handspring for the first time.

"I'm fine, Noah. You should get ready for school."

"No! I'm staying here with you."

"Noah, she's okay," Todd assures him. "Let's get you to school."

"You can't make me. I need to watch her in case she has another seizure."

"Please, honey, I promise I won't get up without Dad here. I'm so proud of you for getting him. That was very responsible."

"You need me here, Mom. That could happen again."

"Noah, it's better for Mom if you go to school," Todd says. I wish he hadn't. I don't want Noah to think I am better off without him. I'm the only mother I know that prays for snow days so I can hang out with my child. Noah does leave, but his long face pains me.

I am expected to shoot an interview for a new film I am exploring in a half hour.

Lying flat on the couch at eight in the morning is not what I intended for today. Last night I organized all my video equipment, loaded my lights into the car, and took my subject's complicated breakfast order that I planned to pick up on my way to her house. I'm still reviewing my gear list and my prepared questions when I say to Todd, "I think I can do the interview. I'm just not sure about unloading the forty-pound light kit."

"You have no obligation. There's no time frame."

"No, but she's expecting me to bring breakfast for her and her family."

"Beth. You're feeling weak. I'm sure she will understand. Want me to call her for you?"

"Would you?"

At what point did I schedule this project, before or after excusing myself from all expectations? The project is all wrong and I know it. My intent to interview other cancer patients to find a connection to their emotions and their disease is too close to my own story.

Todd has left me on the couch wrapped in a blanket. My laptop is on the coffee table a foot away; all I have to do is reach for it. I wonder if I can without passing out. The suggestion of creating a legacy box enters my foggy brain. Am I too weak to organize my photos? No, but the very idea of it is making me nauseous. I feel sorry for the unfortunate person put to the task of preserving them. It's the least I can do to consolidate.

How come this feels like the opposite of a passion project? This compiling of photos might be bittersweet if I were creating a slide show for Noah's bar mitzvah. There is nothing sweet about imagining its premiere at my memorial.

What's really motivating me is my need to control the selection of photos to be enlarged and hung on an easel at my service. Being camera shy and never learning how to pose for a picture has produced some very unphotogenic images. Now, as I review these pictures post-cancer, I have a different take on the same photos I once cringed at.

It is a little too late for a lesson on organizing my digital photos. How much easier it would be if they were all stuffed in shoeboxes. Sifting through thousands of images located in multiple folders containing duplicates with different file sizes is the kind of time-intensive task I despise. Ultimately, willy-nilly, I impulsively trash whole folders I shouldn't have. Goddamn legacy box. Luckily I am not a hoarder, but the photographs and my journals, essays, unfinished screenplays, and stories—I hope nobody takes the time to read through them, but burning them seems, well, odd.

Twenty minutes later I realize this is punitive and as I'm working on releasing myself from expectations, I direct the Mac arrow to Shut Down. What the hell is a legacy box really? There is a stack of photo calendars I created over the last ten years and the leather-bound journal I have been keeping for Noah since his birth. That will have to suffice.

A friend of mine dying of cancer had asked me to help her create a legacy video for her children, a verbal history of her life. We never got to it. Personally, I haven't decided on this type of remembrance. I can picture someone opening my legacy box to find pictures of Noah, a folder of his mementos such as ticket stubs, drawings, school accomplishments, etc., and saying, "She clearly didn't understand what a legacy box is."

In my formative years I was a prolific songwriter and composer, but there is little record of that. There were acting roles in amateur productions; a college degree; a life in New York City; my career editing television commercials for every product from Pampers to Pepsi, with the majority of them preserved on obsolete formats; two unproduced screenplays; a documentary; a family; a home.

Fuck it. I want to *live* my life not spend time making legacy boxes of my unfinished one.

28

NEW YEAR'S EVE

December 31, 2017

Todd, Noah, Tom, and I drive down to Maryland to spend New Year's Eve with my family instead of hosting our annual party. My surgery is January third. By then the hospital should be fully staffed and the anesthesiologist recovered from his hangover. Dr. Kan doesn't seem to be the kind of guy that would tie one on before surgery.

No one expects this New Year's Eve to go down as anything we will want to remember. Though sprawled out on my sister's couch, eating takeout sushi and binge watching something unmemorable is special in its own right. We are asleep by midnight despite our promise to bang pots and pans. What are we looking forward to in 2018, I wonder?

It's 2 a.m. Todd lies asleep next to me in bed; Noah is asleep on a cot. Though there is a separate room for Noah, he has chosen to nest with us. How many times have I watched Noah, like a burglar in the dark, enter our bedroom at home and situate himself for sleep with such resolve? Todd was too tired to complain and I relished it in less than quiet ways. I miss those days.

Tonight I have the honor of hearing both Noah and Todd intermittently shout out unintelligible phrases throughout the night. Their snoring is like the healing sounds of night rain.

The next month I will lie in this room without my two boys, beckoning the memory of their sweet smell, their snores, and my window into their dream lives. I will miss the glow of Todd's cell phone in the middle of the night, and so many other precious reminders of our marriage.

The boys are going back to New York today, the day before my surgery. We have decided it is better for Noah to leave while I look healthy. Have I compromised my needs by not asking Todd to stay? At first I wanted him to be there when I got out of surgery, but then I realized that doesn't prove his loyalty. I am well taken care of and he has responsibilities at home. If this surgery were in New York it would be a different case.

At precisely 10 a.m. Todd efficiently packs the car while I sit on the floor with Noah who is crying as if he's going to miss all the fun.

"No way am I going with Dad. I am staying here with you."

"Honey, you have Tom. You three guys are going to be great."

"Dad is so mean to me. He won't let me do anything. He's always yelling at me."

"Actually it's me that's always yelling at you."

"Yeah, but I love you. I hate my life. I'm willing to give up my childhood and go to work. Skip right over it."

"No. I want you to enjoy your childhood. Oh my gosh, Noah, you only get one."

"I don't care. All children who have a parent die—their childhood is over."

"But I'm going to be fine. I promise I'll be home in no time."

"I can't believe you're making me be alone with Dad."

"And Tom."

"I don't give a shit. Dad's a jerk."

"Noah, just do your work and listen to Dad without getting hysterical. He will have nothing to be angry at. Every time I've been away you guys have worked really well together. He's helping with your homework and he is way more patient than I ever am."

"I don't care, you're fine."

"We can still read together every night. Now that you have your new phone we can FaceTime. I'll order the book today so we can read back and forth. What is it again? Queen Elizabeth of…?

"*Eleanor of Aquitaine: A Biography.*"

"Right, amusing book."

"What?"

"I could read the dictionary with you and it would be fun. Now it's time to go. Dad wants to be home for dinner. Maybe you can convince him to take you out for Mexican. Not to Mexican Kitchen."

Now that Noah's agreed to leave, I want to grab him (and Artemis), enroll Noah in a Maryland school, and send Tom and Todd on their way. Tom's expression is that of a traveler's bittersweet good-bye to one of his favorite ports. His smiling face gives me solace: he will distract Noah, but that doesn't diminish the pain I experience as the car pulls out of the driveway and disappears from view.

* * *

I know there is something I am forgetting to do before tomorrow's surgery. Tomorrow. The tumors in my stomach will be gone. I wonder how many pounds I will lose. How much cancer will be killed in the hunt? Will the tumors grow back like the Demogorgon in the show *Stranger Things*? It's a terrifying show in which the slimy creature with hundreds of tentacles is out to kill. Every time the characters think the Demogorgon is under control, it seeps back in like my metastatic cancer.

Now I remember: the "advance" in "advance directive" means prior to the day of surgery and implies careful consideration. Lucky for me, a person who is pragmatic, parental, conscientious, and bossy (helpful in getting things done) is just down the hall. Karyn's identity makes her the obvious appointee as my agent. It doesn't occur to me she may want to decline, but I assume she will appreciate the trust it takes for me to burden her. At this point in the story my editor is asking, "Where is Todd in all this?" He just left to take care of Noah and Tom and no, we did not discuss any directive at all.

Now that I have reviewed the pre-surgery checklist I remember the oncology educational video that specifies it must be completed prior to my surgical date. One bullet point in the video tells me to build my pelvic floor and deep abdominal muscles. I stopped doing "8 Minute Abs" a year ago and have ignored core workouts in my exercise routine. Crap, I should have watched this a month ago; nevertheless I lie on my back and do a hundred sit-ups until my abdomen spasms. I likely tore a muscle. Perhaps I miscalculated the time it would take to prepare.

29

SURGERY

January 3, 2018

At 8 a.m. the next morning I enter Johns Hopkins, take the elevator to the second floor, and hand over my advance directive. Feeling rather at ease, except for my strained abdominal muscles, I am taken through the preoperative process. Meeting the anesthesiologist is my number one priority. I want to tell him not to give me too much anesthesia, but to make sure I get enough, considering my small size. I suggest he say nice things to me when I'm under and crack a joke every once in a while. Lastly, I want to ask him to leave his cell phone outside the operating room, but I don't want him to think I'm difficult, so I leave the last part out.

The nurse's name is Miriam, my mother's name, which I take as a good sign. Nurse Miriam brings mother Miriam a hospital blanket from the incubator at my request. Repeatedly I tell Mom and Karyn to enjoy the day and come back later. I won't know they are gone. Dr. Kan estimates I will be five hours in the operating theater, which makes me feel like it's my Broadway debut. When it is curtain time, the anesthesiologist goes out of focus and I think I've fallen into the orchestra pit before I black out. When the lights come back up, I am in the recovery room, rambling like a drunken sailor wanting to know if the prairie dogs are okay and why these canines are considered rodents.

The new wing in the hospital has private rooms with windows. There was a slight misunderstanding before the surgery when I tried to make a reservation for room 7 because I heard it had a good view. Apparently they don't do that in hospitals. Anyway, the room is great, the nurses are awesome, and I can push that little button for morphine anytime I want.

When my mom and sisters visit, someone always wants to spend the night and not because the Jell-O is good. However, it is a guilt-free way of watching Netflix all day and it gets pretty exciting waiting for me to move my bowels. I need help getting to the bathroom, so when I have a stool emerge, someone will be there to cheer and pop the champagne. This means I will be out of this joint soon.

The more laps I take around the hallways are also cause for applause. Someone brought me cute slippers for my jaunts. A nurse sees me wearing them as I walk alone pushing my IV pole and yells at me. How would I know they had a fall protection program? The nurse is really pissed, like I am putting her job in jeopardy. She isn't even my nurse. She makes me freeze, take off my slippers, and put on the non-skid pink socks she hands me. It is then I notice large posters through-out the corridor logging the number of falls there have been this week. I almost became a number. I no longer walk the halls unless a family member is with me for protection.

One night, alone in my room, I hear screams. I know from experience a call to the nurse's station isn't the most efficient way of getting attention. They don't just hang around there, that's why patients all have their nurse's cell phones. I don't know who is in more despair than me, so I wait it out. But the scream doesn't cease. I call my nurse's cell and tell her a patient in room 20 needs assistance and quick. A team of nurses arrive swiftly and all is fine. Apparently, the woman couldn't reach her remote.

* * *

I'm not fully repaired. When Dr. Kan visited me this morning I was alone. The man does his rounds at 6 a.m. I feared this moment. Dr. Kan can't find a reason to keep me in the hospital any longer. He is very pleased, in awe really. My recovery has beaten his expectations. He calls me his hero-ine. He feels confident he got everything.

But did you get the anxiety? I want to ask. He can see I am less than thrilled to leave. All the nurses who took care of me during the last six days and considered me brave, now look at a balled-up, shaking woman-child ready for a straitjacket, not freedom. Sure it's easy to be brave in here. What's waiting for me in the real world? Expectations, obsessions, fear of making mistakes about the future.

Minutes from now I will be discharged. I pack my clothes, check the refrigerator down the hall to throw out my leftovers, and steal a few packs of saltines. Sitting on the edge of the bed with the IV still jutting out of my sleeve and bags at my feet, I feel like an orphan with trepidations about my next move. I am frozen except for the tears rambling down my face.

When Mauri and Karyn arrive they take one look at me, one look at each other, and utter, "Oh, Beth." Their voices seem to ache with total understanding. Dropping to either side of me, they allow me to cry generously. "I'm damaged goods. I'm cursed," I declare. They don't say a thing; they just rub my back. "I'm so frightened to walk out of this hospital with no purpose or will to live fully," I moan. "I'm so scared." I fear that without cancer in the immediate foreground my quest to live fully will dissolve. How long, I wonder, before the spiritual transformation I long for is complete? I feel like I'm still on trial. To stand confident in my new freedom, surely I need a lot more time. If I have a long life in front of me, please, God, don't let me be a disappointment.

When I settle down, they push me in a wheelchair toward the hospital exit, and although I am afraid, I feel what it means for people to have my back.

30

WHAT'S HAPPENING
AT HOME

January 9, 2018

Most people I know have a family member look after their kids when they are ill while husband and wife huddle in the shadowy areas of death speaking in hushed lullabies. Some struggle with coordinating their kids' lives from afar, favoring rides to their after-school activities not to mention their therapy sessions. So while I have three sisters and a mother that could look after Noah and our exchange student, Tom, nobody can do it better than Todd.

When I leave the hospital my sisters push me toward the hospital's revolving doors, knowing they will be circling me back in three weeks' time. My life wouldn't be this way without Todd.

This is what's going on in my house right now: composting, recycling, taking care of Noah, Tom, Artemis, and our two cats. Todd is managing four properties, our home, researching health insurance, taking care of his father, setting up our Airbnb, and maintaining our friendships.

*　*　*

When I come home, he gives me the ultimate gift: he does not babysit me or ask if I am okay every moment. We have typical discussions, routine days, and after he tells me how exhausted he is from waking early and preparing the boys' breakfast and lunch, I pick up my slack of forgotten responsibilities. He makes me forget I have cancer. Cancer does not stop us from annoying one another, however. It doesn't stop Todd from getting irritated when I shut the door too hard therefore compromising the hinge, or forgetting to fill the cat's dry food, or by how I don't organize the dishwasher in the way that makes sense to him. But to see Todd's same expression of placid impatience reassures me that I am not feeble. Cancer is also like an indiscretion Todd and I choose to live with and not address. We don't plan on going our separate ways and it doesn't help to dwell on the elephant in the room.

Nevertheless, illness has created stress for Todd. Every twenty-one days I receive treatment in DC and during that time Todd runs our house like a well-oiled machine. When I return I disrupt his system and then leave again. One of my sisters or Mom want to escort me home, which I know makes Todd anxious. Even though they come to care for me, I inevitably want to cater to them.

Karyn drives me home after a week in Maryland and on the way I call Todd to sheepishly ask if he could change the sheets in the guest room and perhaps vacuum. This man has so many obligations and I'm putting yet another thing on his to-do list. Karyn is coming to help and yet I'm worried about the amount of pillows on her bed and whether there is almond milk in the refrigerator. My compulsion to host is steeped in my need for control. Getting care in Maryland was the best choice for all of us, because had my treatments been in New York, our house would have turned into an inn and my marriage would possibly have unraveled. Not to say Todd doesn't love my family, he does, but we all have our limits.

Todd is my glue. He gives me the home-field advantage. He may not always be in every scene in my story, but he is the engine. You don't have to see it to know it's working.

31

FACETIME

January 5, 2018

Noah's seventh grade class is studying the Italian Renaissance and reading *Queen Eleanor, Independent Spirit of the Medieval World: A Biography of Eleanor of Aquitaine.* The book is as difficult as the title predicts. I promised Noah that even though I was in Maryland we could take turns reading it.

When my FaceTime rings I am on the ready to tap Accept. I am still surprised by this technology. Noah's gorgeous face fills the screen. For what feels like several quiet minutes we both tilt our heads at different angles, soaking in the essence of the other. Noah lies on his back in his bed. I spy his beloved blanket, the one I gave him at birth, tucked beside him.

I have not yet received my edition of the book, which I had to track down from a rare bookstore. In the meantime, Noah will hold his copy to the iPhone camera so I can read my portion. "Are you ready?" I ask.

"Wait, I got it somewhere." He holds the phone with his face so that my end goes dark. I feel like I'm in heavy turbulence as his phone whirls around the room, Noah coming in and out of the shot.

"Noah, put the phone down."

"Wait I'm almost—shit…" I hear objects knocking around.

"Noah?"

His pointer finger fills the frame signaling one minute. Then he replaces the finger with a close-up of his goofy expression. He is so silly and I love this, but it might go on for hours.

"Honey?"

"Okay, okay. I got it. Artemis, Artemis." He is calling for the dog. "Come here, buddy. Come on." Noah pushes Artemis's square head and disoriented puppy eyes to the camera.

"Noah, please…"

"Fine." He holds the page to the iPhone camera; the page goes in and out of focus.

"'Sitting beside Louis at the high table, Eleanor presided over the wedding feast with an ease and a style beyond her fifteen years, seeing that…'"

"Got to go, Mom. Dad's calling me for dinner."

And with that I sense Noah is all right. When I am home Noah lingers and ignores our calls to the table; tonight he dutifully responds to Todd. "It's dinnertime, got to go!" Five words that I am actually grateful to hear.

32

MOM STEALS THE SHOW

January 10, 2018

I planned to write and meditate during my recuperation at Karyn's house. What better opportunity to be on a retreat and alone with my thoughts? But respecting privacy isn't something my family of origin does well. Knowing what's best for one another, we appear in each other's kitchens without notice. My fantasy of the bedroom on the second floor of Karyn's house as my ashram isn't logical. With Starbucks and Bagel Maven minutes away, and four eager people competing to serve me, I have a lot of company. Besides, as most of my fantasies go, the allure of a meditation retreat lost its appeal after I played out the experience in my head.

Anyone who has ever met my mom, even if just for a moment, recognizes her strength, enthusiasm, and all-out optimism. The woman is either doing yoga, Rollerblading, or taking a dance class every day of the week, visiting someone in need, or showing up for all her daughters' and grandchildren's events while caring for her husband. Her constitution goes unmatched. I'll call her one day and ask, "How's everything?"

"Fine. Everything's great." She coughs. "It was a beautiful sunrise yoga practice. Our regular teacher didn't show up, so I taught the class."

"How's everything?" I ask the next day.

"Oh, so much better than yesterday."

"Yesterday you said you were great?"

"I had a sore throat. I spent most of the day in bed, but I feel like a different person today. It's not a cold." It pains me to see her blow her nose or rub her cheekbone to suppress a sinus headache, but no matter how many times I ask, she never admits to discomfort.

Before I went for surgery on January third, she was downplaying a bulge the size of a pebble in her neck. She would admit the area was tender, but not a problem. Mom spent two nights sleeping in my hospital room curled up in a chair when she could have used the pull-out couch. During that time the lump in her neck grew to the size of a golf ball. No matter how many episodes of *The Marvelous Mrs. Maisel* we watched, she could no longer ignore the pain. The nurse began to bring Mom aspirin every time she gave me my meds.

By the time I left the hospital my mom's lump was still growing and undiagnosed. We took guesses. A very large tonsil stone? A tumor? We now had a new family drama and scrambled for doctors and tests to be ordered.

Meanwhile I was taken to Karyn's to convalesce and begin my anticipated retreat. Everyone's focus had shifted to my mom's health; no longer was my water being refilled every five minutes. I think I'll have privacy after all, I thought, but under the circumstances the anticipated quiet was disconcerting.

* * *

Coming out of my Dilaudid-induced fog, I hear commotion coming from the stairway. My sisters appear on opposite sides of my frail mom, propping her up. They lead her to the other side of my sick bed. It doesn't take me long to realize I have a roommate in my infirmary.

Mom exceeds me in the pain department. How this mysterious protruding bump in her neck can be more agonizing than my surgery is beyond imagination. But it is big. The doctors instruct Mom to drink a lot of water, suck on lemon drops, and take antibiotics—all intolerable for her. She thinks a chai latte counts as both her nourishment and hydration for the day.

* * *

If I feel acute pain from the glue holding my stomach together, I keep it to myself. As Mom sleeps, I shift positions quietly, not wanting to wake her. Mom's always cold so I give her my extra blankets in the middle of the night; besides, I'm having hot flashes. In the morning Karyn routinely delivers me a beautiful plate of scrambled eggs with sliced avocado in bed. I eat discretely, afraid the sight of food will disgust my mom. She doesn't like food, not on a normal day, let alone on a day she's in pain.

For Mom, swallowing a pill is a very big obstacle. It gets lodged in her throat. We try creative approaches to get her to swallow. Everything is a guessing game. We open her prescribed antibiotic capsule and sprinkle its contents onto a spoonful of vanilla ice cream. Whenever it's time to take her medication the room transforms into an ER with two or three people leaning over her holding water, the spoon, and a piece of bread to make sure the medicine will stay down. I watch this tense operation from my side of the bed feeling like the patient who should have been discharged days ago.

At one point my mom is in excruciating pain, so Jill suggests I give her one of my Dilaudids. I become an accomplice when I hand Mom a two-milligram tablet of the narcotic. Mom and I both weigh in at eighty pounds and I assume she can handle two milligrams if it takes me four to feel its effects. We assure her relief is on the way. Instead, an ambulance is on its way. Mom is hallucinating, her dizziness insufferable. There is no way she can make it downstairs with her equilibrium as it is. The paramedics remove her from the bed and strap her into a medical chair. The route down the stairs is so precarious I think we all will have heart attacks. Please don't drop Mom over the banister. The wheels of the chair bump on every step and I ache for her.

Transferring Mom from the chair to the gurney and then into the ambulance leaves me lonely. I miss our shared sick bed. I would gladly trade my meditation time for another second lying next to my mom. The paramedics whisk Mom away; my sisters follow. I am left behind watching this surreal episode unfold. I am her petrified child without any instructions on what to do next. It occurs to me that soon Noah might witness an incident identical to this one, only it will be me carted away and Noah left in bewilderment wondering if this is the last time he will see his mother.

* * *

Mauri calls to tell me disaster has been averted, though we almost killed my mother. They admitted her into the overcrowded hospital where she spends twelve hours in the hallway, though they immediately give her fluids and anti-biotics through an IV. The doctor says all the medications she was taking without food were wrecking her system. On top of that we never should have opened the antibiotic capsules. It erodes the esophagus and doesn't allow it to do its job. Finally, the narcotic Dilaudid is the strongest out there. Asking where she got it, they were not the least bit surprised it came from her cancer-stricken daughter who recently underwent major surgery.

* * *

Mom entered my hospital room on January third with a cat-egory-one swollen gland. By the time I was discharged she had a golf ball–sized lump that was category two. When she was moved into my infirmary at Karyn's, it was category three and by the time I poisoned her with Dilaudid and opened the capsule exposing her to the carcinogenic drug particles, she was category four. Mom's sympathy pains turned out to be a clogged salivary gland. Turns out I got my privacy after all, but I definitely didn't get any peace of mind.

33

I CAN'T LIVE
WITHOUT YOU

February 1, 2018

It took some convincing, but I am flying home alone after my fifth chemotherapy in DC. It was as if the police pulled me over and made me walk a straight line. I passed. The terminal's automatic doors open, I step through, and give one last wave to my mom, who is biting her nail in the car as she strains her neck to see me go.

Once through security, I grab my bags but feel dizzy. My gate is thirty-seven away from where I stand. Fainting would definitely ruin my chances of ever traveling alone after chemotherapy. I flag down an airport golf cart zooming by me.

Todd picks me up from the airport and hands me a beautiful, light and fluffy, seriously melt-in-your-mouth glazed donut. I chew slowly, engrossed in the pleasure a donut can bring, especially if you haven't had one in twenty years. Denial is bullshit. I can say this with authority after months of living with cancer. This donut is a symbol, like the promise of a wedding ring. I vow to love and cherish my cravings.

My first few days home I hang in the background like a visiting aunt, curious, but not wanting to get in the way of an established routine. I am the ousted incumbent. Todd's term is going well. Well, in terms of structure, discipline, and values inherent in military school. It's only a matter of time before my reentry and bad influence emboldens Noah to go AWOL. I'm not sure which is the bigger stressor for Todd: my appearance or my absence.

Todd seems to be condemned to drudgery, waking up early to get both boys breakfast, make lunch, and get them out the door only to later prepare dinner. Which leaves him time to manage our recent real estate investments, take care of our home, pick up from after-school activities, and cross-check my medical bills that look like grocery receipts for a family of ten.

Tom greets me with a giant hug, as does Noah along with requests to come see all his new accomplishments. Artemis seems to care less. Noah carries my bag upstairs and wants to help me unpack. In between Noah's excited dialogue, I hear clanging pots in the kitchen. Todd: what is he feeling?

Noah wants to know what the doctors say. I give the Pac-Man analogy, but he wants medical terms. He tells me he's been doing a lot of research on marijuana and is binge watching a TV comedy series, *Disjointed*, about a cannabis dispensary in Los Angeles. Watching Kathy Bates light up a joint on prime-time TV has opened the gates. The behavior normalizes getting high and although the characters act stoned, it looks like a lot of fun. I can smell the bong water from where I'm sitting and assume Noah's binge watching the show isn't a good sign.

I make a decision to all watch a show together, but something besides *Disjointed*. Our bedroom becomes a salon for our screenings. Noah lies with me on the bed, Tom on the chaise longue to my right, and Artemis at the foot of the bed. We have chosen to watch *Stranger Things,* a mystery with terrifying supernatural forces with multiple seasons. We start a second episode even though it's nine o'clock. I know the boys will be piling into my bedroom every night to get through at least one season. Todd rarely joins us and I wonder why our screams and laughter isn't more inviting. It doesn't occur to me he may want the room to himself to watch his own program or that he might want to spend some alone time with me.

* * *

When Noah was six he asked me, "Mom, is there anything broken in the world that can't be fixed?" It still throws me today. How can I ease the fears of a boy threatened by his mother's disease? I want to tell him my cancer will go away, instead I tell him how much I love him.

"I'll kill myself if you die," he says flatly.

"I understand, Noah. I couldn't live without you." That was not very well thought out. I basically gave him permission to off himself.

Noah is old enough to get himself to bed, but I cuddle beside him until I am kicked out. Todd is already in bed and I should go to him. Breathing Noah in for one last moment is heartbreaking, because I wish I could stay like this forever. I remember Noah at age eleven being upset about something right before bed. As I got up to leave he said, "Mom, stay here with my feelings." It wasn't that long ago, I tell myself, so I lie back down with him now, keeping his feelings company.

34

RADIOLOGY FRIENDS

A nurse escorts me into the waiting room where I join a small group of characters, advanced in their years, already settled in. We are all in the holding cell before our impending CT scan. I am now very familiar with the cocktail the others are holding: barium. One look at someone drinking it and you know it's unpleasant. Barium dye contrast materials coat the lining of your insides so it can be seen by the X-ray. Anything this difficult to get down better do something amazing. The manufacturers of this toxin have the nerve to brand it as a "smoothie" on the label.

I raise my bottle to my neighbors, a toast to our shared misery. They smile, eager to chat, so I grab off the stack of magazines and bury my head in a *Newsweek*. The ninety-four-year-old man (he told me) likes my idea and rises to peruse the magazines. *Woman's Day, Elle, Vogue,* and

Redbook are the only choices left. He looks defeated so I offer him mine. I know a conversation will ensue and clearly I have given him an opening. Apparently he no longer gets off on the sexual images advertised in those publications. He writes memoirs, science fiction, and speeches for IBM executives. He likes the retirement community he lives in and has been in remission for over twenty years. If I didn't know any better I'd think this is a welcome outing for him. This man emanates happiness. I can't help but think that in comparison to me, he is way ahead of the game.

The woman across from me seems to be struggling to get her "smoothie" down. Unfortunately her daughter couldn't make it to the appointment, because she has a life a thousand miles away. I form a pact with the woman to take a large slurp of barium whenever she does. My suggestion is to drink through a straw and take in three of the biggest sips she can handle. Lower the bottle, take a few deep breaths, and on an inhale repeat the process until all twenty ounces are drained. It must be downed in an hour and while I have seen men literally chug theirs, I need the fully allotted time.

Another man, also much older than I, sits in a wheelchair. His unmanageable beard and steely eyes intimidate me. The two of us are the only ones left in the waiting room. A nurse pops her head in. "Hello, Mr. Kruger, I'll be right back with your drink."

"That's okay, honey, I'm not going to drink."

"Why is that? You know you have to. I'll be right back."

He address me. "She's not going to make me drink it."

"Isn't the CT scan useless without it?" I ask. His look

suggests he isn't having any of this CT scan nonsense and that I'm a fool to drink the stuff. The nurse comes back in, opens the seal, punctures it with a bendy straw, and hands it to him. He dismisses it.

"Mr. Kruger, you have to."

"No, I don't." It's a standoff. She gives him a minute to acquiesce. "I'm just drinking to here." He moves his finger an inch below the top.

The nurse presses, "Oh come on, Mr. Kruger."

"I'll drink a third, but that's it." It is agreed upon and the nurse leaves us alone. He seems so resigned to death I wonder why he is here for a scan in the first place. As if he read my mind, he says, "Pancreatic cancer. I was told I had six months to live, but that was reduced to three once they found a giant spot on my right lung." He is completely at ease, even boastful of his end-of-life arrangements. I learn his wife is housebound due to her oxygen tanks and is his only dependent. His son is grown. She will be financially comfortable with the one hundred and fifty thousand dollars collected from his three life insurance policies.

"Body donation, that's the way to go. I got this friend who told me about it and I gave a call up to Albany Medical Center." Donating his body to research at the medical center will take care of all his financial responsibilities including transportation and cremation. This sounds good, an all-expense paid trip to the afterlife. This, he tells me, is called their "Anatomical Gift Program." I am seriously honored that he is sharing this information with me. He seems concerned for my end-of-life plans too. He gives me the name of his contact person at the medical center.

Though I don't write it down, I thank him. His barium doesn't look like it's a third down, but I don't see why it's worth his discomfort at this point. I check my watch and take the last swig of my barium as I hear, "Miss Cramer, it's time for your CT scan."

35

PLAYING THE C CARD

Cancer affects people in strange ways that I might not have recognized were I not the patient. Snippets of my eulogy are being written on Facebook. Family posts photographs of me as a baby.

"Remember this one!"

Those slideshows coming into my feed give me a strong feeling that my time is limited.

Having my picture taken surreptitiously and at inopportune moments seem calculated: me on the phone, me putting bread in the toaster, me in bed writing with my beady eyes under the wool hat that will forever be associated with my cancer story.

While I had no intention of playing the C card too quickly, others wasted no time. A parent of my son's friend was talking to me on her cell phone while driving.

We were arranging a play date when she got pulled over by the police. I heard her drop the phone; she had forgotten I was still on the line. After the discourse, "License and registration. Do you know why I pulled you over?" etc., the woman confessed that while she was guilty, her friend who she was talking to had cancer. She still got a ticket.

In her defense, I once took my friend to a chemotherapy appointment and got pulled over for not minding a yield sign. I told the officer my friend was late for chemotherapy. He gave us an escort to the medical building.

Using the C card mortified me, until I found myself using it. Having no ulterior motive, I told my optometrist that I had stage 4 cancer the day before my appointment. He didn't charge me for the visit. Telling people wasn't high on my agenda, not the bank tellers, my barista, my yoga teachers, or good acquaintances. Later I found the C card useful for getting full refunds on canceled tickets and travel, even late fees. Should a police officer pull me over for speeding, I have already formulated a plan to take off my cap and reveal my bald head for sympathy and hopefully be let off with a warning.

Hesitant to wear a scarf or reveal my baldness was holding me back from playing the C card harder. There is a learning curve to cancer. For instance, I wore my wig to a hot yoga class. Ten minutes into the class I crept out of the room and came back with my head exposed. I felt humiliated for wearing a wig in a 120-degree room when everyone in the studio knew I was bald. But once I got over being self-conscious, my practice improved and I had a deeper spiritual experience.

Standing in line at our local bakery, impatient and concerned that the woman in front of me would take the last honey grain roll, I almost wished I had not worn my wig—maybe pity would move me to the front of the line. By the way I also wish, completely separate from the cancer, that people would know what they want to order before it becomes their turn. Someone told me cancer would make the little things no longer matter, but I can't seem to get past this one.

Anyway, it is hot in the bakery and beads of sweat are accumulating at my hairline, making my wig loosen, resulting in a very large forehead effect. This happens also when someone hugs me and inevitably catches a strand of hair that pulls the whole wig back. I get anxious when someone comes at me with arms outstretched.

There is no benefit to losing your hair and having a shortened lifespan. I would like to petition for a cancer membership card much like AAA that give discounts for movies, expedited check-in and -out of DMV and airport security, and Starbucks refills. It will be several years before I can take advantage of senior citizen discounts. My IRA has a healthy amount of savings so shouldn't I be able to withdraw without penalty?

An upcoming chemotherapy session is scheduled for the end of day, a very unfavorable time slot. Looking for a persuasive reason to be given priority, I hit a roadblock: a cancer center is the one place you can't play the C card.

36

HAVE A GREAT DAY

Most days I woke, fed the dog, took Noah to school, and meditated. This got me to 9 a.m. Lunch was exactly at 11:30 and designated free time to pitch ideas to myself. The list included: write five hundred words a day, read a new book, learn a new instrument, find a new recipe, go grocery shopping, and prepare a dinner to surprise Todd. God, I missed working and the luxury to complain about its pitfalls. The first time I heard someone say on a ski lift, "No one ever goes to his grave saying I wish I worked more," I thought: *not me.* Cancer has been the antidote to a void I challenged myself to fill—with a lot of doubt. Now, my desire is simple: to find beauty in every moment—ultimately.

For meditation this morning I decide to work with a Sankalpa, a mantra. It took a while to settle on one. "I am…enough." Not satisfied, I persist: "I am…happy." No.

"I am…all that is." It's been overused. "I am…" My dog yawns, distracting me. His exaggerated tongue makes no apology. This strikes me as comical and suddenly I have my mantra to manifest my deepest heartfelt desire: "I am in the moment." Setting my meditation timer for five minutes, I end twenty seconds early, telling myself it's superfluous to wait for the chime. Old habits die hard.

This morning I promise Todd I will do some weeding around the yard. I can feel his tension mounting every time he walks outside. He's in and out of town fixing faucets, unclogging toilets, and painting offices in our rental properties, and every time he gets home, he pulls weeds on the way to the front door. Oh the guilt I have mounted from seeing him hunched over a bed of hostas, the white plastic bucket he gets from Lowe's between his legs, as he tweezes out the weed's root. The heat shows no mercy and the wrath of an angry homeowner whose wife is inside meditating on getting well seeps into my energy field.

Todd teases that I am always surprised by how great the garden looks, as if it is magically maintained. As I fork the dirt to unearth a root, I find myself at ease. Soon I am hauling barrels of mulch around the property until the mulch mountain lessens. This does not feel like avoidance. Later I recognize there is no fixation or recrimination for not accomplishing something noteworthy. Weeding was just something I was doing, the weather was nice, and Todd was within earshot.

Think of all the days I could have spent weeding over the past years, relieving Todd of the burden. If only I'd had this perspective. Instead, weeds weren't a good enough task. I would have rather sat and done nothing. Now I reflect on what was keeping me stuck: weeding was a metaphor for failure and a reminder that I had nothing better going on.

Months ago, before cancer, I would have said a day of doing nothing for me is a hole, not an open sky. When I lean on nothing, more nothing follows until something materializes. Hopes are raised and then the something falls apart, revealing it was nothing all along. All I ever really accomplished was being incredibly self-involved.

One day when I was leaving the hospital after a treatment, a valet held the door for me and said, "Have a great day!" Exhausted and terrified, I almost missed this. His words could have pissed me off. How am I going to have a great day? I have cancer. Instead, I lifted my eyes to his and smiled. It was as if he were a wise shaman, giving me a universal truth in the way of a proverb: "Have a great day."

37

FUCK IT

It seemed like a positive message to give myself. "Fuck it" is confirmation that I've made it to the other side of compromise. It didn't occur to me that resentment is implied by those words. My husband doesn't want to travel with me? Fuck it. That pair of shoes is too expensive? Fuck it. I really shouldn't drink that second glass of wine. Fuck it.

It is more a retaliation to life than an awakening.

Now that I'm told death is close, it is imperative that I take initiative to go any direction away from stuck. My experience of finding out I have cancer didn't involve anger. What are the five stages of grief? Denial, anger, bargaining, depression, and acceptance? I went right to acceptance, or so I thought.

The only pity I have is how much I missed when allegedly I was living in hell. Had I only said fuck it the last thirty years, I might not have grown a fucking tumor. Oops, there is it. Anger.

I don't talk about anger a lot. The therapist who told me to speak my truth wasn't specific as to how, or what, but she was clear as to whom. Here's the question: How does it make others feel when they are the reason for my "Fuck it" response? From my side of the story, those two words are a more concise version of, *It's fine you don't want to do what I do, I love you anyway, but I'm going for it.* They might hear, *Fuck it, you shit, you are letting me down again and forcing me to do this thing I don't know if I really want to do alone.* "Fuck it" should be reserved for situations when I'm flying solo.

People tell me they are impressed by the way I'm dealing with cancer, as if I'm doing it in style. All I'm doing is acting like I don't have it. Uh-oh, a realization. I might be hovering over the first stage of grief. Anyhow, my fuck it routine has set an example. It's a real compliment when someone with cancer tells me I inspire them.

I am no one's role model. I didn't have a cancer role model and I know for absolute sure there will never be one. My way of dealing with the reality of doctors' appointments and treatments is to make it fiction. I use the novel I started and get into character. Isa. At least in the beginning, I used Isa to run offense as I stood in the background taking notes. I was so focused on the material I needed for the book that I had my *team* pay attention to the doctor's protocol and advice, while I studied his gestures and facial expressions for the novel or novel-turned-screenplay, if I'm lucky.

I intended to hide my cancer, but eventually I found myself just letting it loose. When the yoga instructor asks at the beginning of the class: *Does anyone have any injuries?*

I raise my hand and blurt out, *I have cancer!* I saw a new massage therapist recently and was given a health form to fill out. *Are you currently taking any medication?* I try to recall the names of all five, but put down two. *Are you currently seeing a health-care professional?* Yes. *Please list reason for treatment.* I start to write Canc—then recoil. *What? Why?* Will the therapist become alarmed once she sees that *word* on my form? Will the easy smile of someone expecting to do an ordinary sports massage shift to intense concern in treating a cancer patient? Has she done cancer massages before if that's such a thing? Do I think she will touch me with kid gloves? The fact that I have cancer is irrelevant to my massage. I'm not there for cancer management, I'm there because I practiced my tennis serve for two hours straight and my shoulder is killing me.

I leave the rest of the form blank and sign my name. The amount of times I have given my signature has increased at least 50 percent since September 2017; so has my speed. With just two quick strokes I get ready to collect relief. When the massage therapist reaches my Mediport, I remember: cancer doesn't let me get away with anything.

Giving myself permission to choose what I needed previously meant not taking others into consideration. Acting impulsively seemed merely foolish; looking for new opportunities felt too late. Somehow, I can't explain why, facing death makes "too late" sound irrational. Impending death let me feel off the hook initially. If it hasn't been my time in the past, now surely is. It's not selfish, foolish, or too late when time is limited. Too late is too late if you believe such a thing exists as I did, pre cancer. Too late gets really magnified when the game's almost over.

Should we all say fuck it more, regardless of life span? I'm not advising it. We collectively can't. Why? Too many of us will be around for a long time and that's a long time for people to hate us, to resent us, and label us selfish. I can afford to fuck it because when people are told I am going to die they let my self-interest slide. There is no end to the usage of the phrase, "Fuck it" when you have cancer. If I'm feeling really needy I'll use the C word and fuck it in one sentence. *If I didn't have cancer I wouldn't ask for vacation, but fuck it, this is my time.* Using both is completely unnecessary. The receiver of the C word reacts with a fuck it response anyway. If I said, though I never would, *Can I please have that last piece of pie?* the person I ask would say, *Oh fuck it, go ahead even though I wanted it.*

It makes me feel bold just to say fuck it. When I say it, I sound serious. Even I believe I'm going to follow through. The force and tinge of obscenity has a laxative affect. People believe I'm really going for it, whatever it is. Other people who hear me say fuck it, start parroting me as if I coined the phrase or it was our sorority pledge.

I'm dying to live, but some days I'm just dying and living. Living with cancer. Dying in a few years, give or take. On those days fuck it just seems appropriate.

38

CYCLE FOR SURVIVAL

March 11, 2018

I don't want to go. I want to say ***fuck it***. The last thing I want is to be a poster child for cancer. Cycle for Survival's indoor team cycling event raises funds given to Sloan Kettering for rare cancer research. It is an incredibly successful event that started in New York and now takes place at hundreds of gyms across the country. For the past seven years I rode in New York for other people fighting cancer; this year I have cancer and will step up as the team mascot.

We cycle in teams: Team Perry, Team Rockstar, Linn4survival, Tough as Nails, and our team, Positivity. The event looks like this: music pumps, young millennials on stationary bikes sweat while team members dance and cheer. Of course there is a lot of pom-pom waving. Several seductive instructors on a riser keep the energy going.

"Get up off the saddle, push harder and harder. Dial up the resistance and let's show cancer who's boss."

Teams in varying swag with logos stating whom they ride for are doing something, anything to make a difference. In between sets, of which there are four, a cancer survivor takes the stage to tell their story.

"I was told I had two months to live. Thanks to my niece who started Team Greg and all the donations given to Sloan Kettering, I am here with you today celebrating, five years later."

Who do I ride in honor of? Since my first cycle in 2012, I didn't have any friends or family with cancer. I was riding for the benefit of cancer research worldwide. In 2013, it hit closer to home. My first friend was diagnosed with a rare cancer and we rode in her honor. In 2014, four friends were diagnosed with four different cancers. In 2015, two of them passed away. I was able to fund-raise with greater intensity in the wake of my new connection to cancer.

Not in a million years would I have imagined myself part of this epidemic. Todd and I are uncomfortable asking friends to donate while they struggle with their own finances. "Team Positivity" was just starting to fund-raise for 2018 when I was diagnosed. What a perfect device for generating donations. Truthfully, I sensed pressure to use myself as a ploy. It would have been easy not to attend Cycle for Survival that year since I'd had surgery two months before the event. I couldn't bring myself to fund-raise, but I did allow my family to send out emails. Family, friends, and relatives gave generously.

While donations were being made under my name, there was something troubling me. The research oncologist at Johns Hopkins told me it was very unlikely a promising trial would be developed in time for me.

When writing *The Isa Stories,* I knew there would be a chapter dedicated to her experience with Cycle for Survival. Isa was perhaps an amalgam of all the women I knew that had cancer, but when I look back at this fictional account, I realize how much it foreshadowed my own feelings.

Isa has reached her summit, the insurmountable. Her friends were there to celebrate her battle. God, that word irks her. It annoys her to hear the term "fighting" cancer. It implies that you are a loser. She realizes how many ways cancer will do that. She fought like hell, went several rounds with chemo, had the operation to remove her ovaries, vomited with the promise of revenge, and this is her party. The thirty thousand dollars her team raised for rare cancer with Isa as their mascot was a success.

She should feel appreciative instead of belittled, Isa told herself. A part of her wished all the contributions her friends and family made on her behalf went into a personal account to fund her bucket list. Treatments were expensive and travel was too much of a luxury. Besides, the charity wasn't likely to help Isa. Trials for ovarian cancer still had a long way to go. How selfish, *she thought,* I'm not a good person. *Just the thought of it made her cringe with her own greed. But she also knew all those people would probably have loved to give money directly to her. People are always asking what they can do. People register for baby showers and weddings, why not end of life occasions?*

After my initial reaction, which was just like Isa's, I decided to attend the event. I had no physical excuse; two months after surgery I could ride a stationary bike no problem. It was not without trepidation, however; I didn't want people cheering for me as a cancer patient. I didn't even want anyone doing something directly for me. For the human species, but not for me, please.

* * *

Noah and Todd joined me and Noah was more than enthusiastic to cycle. Once I could overlook the event photographer stalking me and surreptitiously snapping photos of me with the telltale bandana head covering, I learned something about the event I hadn't thought of: it brought Noah hope. I saw it in his eyes. He says it was his favorite event of the year and he now wears his Cycle for Survival T-shirt with pride.

We are a worldwide community tied together in one way or another by cancer. The event didn't sadden Noah like I'd feared. The positive faces, the music, the money pouring in, and the numbers moving upward on the LED ticker tape above us assured him that we are not alone.

39

SEVENTH AND
FINAL INFUSION

March 13, 2018

I step off the plane, guns a-blazing, at whom I am not sure. I am keenly aware of the big chip on my shoulder. It is my seventh and last chemotherapy. It's the same old routine. I am picked up at the airport, driven to Karyn's, the family descends, and straws are drawn for who will accompany me to chemo the next day. I am two seconds away from biting someone's head off for just moving my water glass. Despite my plea not to be babysat during chemo, someone is coming.

My mother deserves the honor and although I am hesitant, it is impossible for me to deny her this privilege. I would want to be there for Noah. She picks me up early in the morning, offers me snacks, smiles, and comfort. I am like Jack Nicholson in *The Shining*, descending into madness.

* * *

All I want to do is put on my headphones, listen to my meditation music, and fall asleep. My mom curls into an armchair in the small infusion room with her book and promises to be quiet. To walk around the room takes careful planning: roll the IV pole to the side, step over the power cable, lower the footrest. Everything is annoying me today. So what if it's a small room? Mom doesn't take up a lot of space. I want her to be warm and the room temperature is cold; this disturbs me. She brought three blankets and won't take one for herself. She keeps tucking one of them around my legs. Maybe that is it—even in the moment I don't know what sets me off—but I turn fierce. In what I can only imagine is the voice coming from someone un-hinged, I command my mother to leave the room. She does.

Now I cannot meditate, I am too busy berating myself for my behavior. I grab my phone and text Karyn:

I just yelled at Mom to get out of the room. She is some-where in the hospital, probably devastated. Please come and be with her. I feel so bad. I am such an asshole.

I text Mauri:

Please come to the hospital. I need you to be with Mom. I just yelled at her and I am sure she feels awful. I am so so sorry.

I text Jill:

Check to see if Mauri or Karyn is coming to the hospital. I yelled at Mom and need someone to come over here and do damage control.

Then I text Todd:

If you were here I would feel guilty if I yelled at you, but I yelled at my mom and I can't live with myself. Where the hell are you when I need you? I know, home taking care of the boys. I love you!

Finally, I text Mom and beg her to come back into the room. I tell Mom I should have never, ever allowed her to come with me today. I knew there was a chance that who-ever was near me would be a target. Fucking cancer.

40

MOST WANTED

March 30, 2018

Nonstop, preferred airport, three tickets on the exact dates wanted. When I advance to seat assignments on the website, I accept the challenge even with the dissonance playing out in my head. A window and an aisle seat for Tom and Noah and one for myself a row behind. Sadly I will have a stranger as my neighbor instead of Todd, who has chosen to stay behind. Hastily, I select "no" to travel insurance; that tap is the sound of death. For one heart-stopping moment I consider Todd, the cost, my health, but then I swallow the moon and click confirm. The final screen might as well have read GOOD LUCK! Instead of CONFIRMED.

Todd drops us at the airport. Todd, the passionate skier and snowboarder, the one who makes sure I am dressed in proper layers, who wipes snow out of my glove after a fall, and who finds nirvana making beautiful turns down the mountain and from all-you-can-eat wings at après-ski, is really staying home with Artemis. One week after my seventh and final chemotherapy treatment, I check in three bags, one six-foot wheeled ski bag, three boot bags, and two teenagers at the airport kiosk.

It is spring break for Noah and Tom and we hope to catch some fresh powder in Vail, Colorado where Mauri and my brother-in-law, Keith, will host us at their ski house for a week. Besides altitude sickness, nothing is going to keep me from snowboarding.

Walking with my friend Alan, I asked, "Do you think I am different after cancer then I was before?"

"Definitely. You're absolute."

Mauri arranged a driver to pick us up at the airport and take us the two hours into Vail. I didn't want a driver, but this is how it goes when loved ones worry. And it was a good thing she did. After getting into the town car, I realized my wallet was lost in an airport.

* * *

Being in Colorado, it is my duty to visit a weed dispensary. On the wall is a chart: "Know Your Medicine." I purchase five buds of something that claims to inhibit cell growth in tumors and cancer cells. The day before we leave, I walk into a UPS store, pack the buds in nothing much more than a padded mailer, and address it to myself in New York. I'm not so naïve that I would bring it on the plane.

Weeks go by and no delivery of my "medicine" has been made. My tracking number is lost, so I decide to call the UPS store against Todd's advice. Luckily I know exactly the day I shipped it and how much it cost. This will easily help them find it.

The woman who picks up the phone sounds familiar to the one I spoke to the day I was there. "I'm hoping you can look in your computer and tell me the tracking number for a package I sent."

"Do you know the date?"

"Yes, and I think you were there. It was just before you were closing. I was with my sister who talks a lot and had her little dog with her." People always remember Mauri; I thought this might help jog the woman's memory. "It was shipped on April second and it cost thirteen dollars and fifty-nine cents." I can hear her typing.

"Ma'am. That package is still here."

"Really?"

"It never left, ma'am. It reeks of pot."

"Oh, shit. Well, can I have my sister come pick it up?"

"We have to discard it."

"Well, why did you keep it then?"

"We are not allowed to touch it. We wait for someone to call and claim it."

"Then what?"

"Most people give fake phone numbers," she says. I don't understand what that has to do with my predicament.

"So I'll have my sister get it," I continue.

"Ma'am, I am underage. I'll get in major trouble if I touch it."

"You don't have to."

"I have a baby at home, I am not going to take any chances of getting arrested."

"So what happens?"

"The cops have to come and dispose of it."

"You won't give them my name, will you?" I remember my name and address on the package as both sender and receiver. "I don't know what the police do, ma'am. It is a federal offense to ship marijuana across state lines." Damn, she was so nice when I was in the store.

Despite losing my wallet somewhere in the airport and becoming most wanted by the Colorado police, I passed the threshold from uncertainty into action. The Transportation Security found my license and I assume I can talk my way out of anything by playing the C card, including my ignorance about federal laws. The certified mail notices that keep showing up at my house remain a mystery, but Todd says I shouldn't claim it. A certified letter is unlikely to be good and based on my decision to notify the postal service that I unsuccessfully tried to smuggle marijuana across state lines may have something to do with it

What lessons have I learned? Get my medical marijuana license in my state, stop thinking I need marijuana to treat cancer, and carry a purse instead of stuffing my wallet in one jacket pocket and my phone in the other. When in doubt, blame everything on cancer.

41

RESULTS

April 5, 2018

Back to Maryland for a CT scan. As Noah plainly put it, "The CT scan to end all CT scans." The results from a seven-month culmination of treatments, including seven cycles of chemotherapy and a major surgery, were about to be revealed. There is nothing like the suspense of a horror movie ending.

It is going to be a stressful day so my sisters ask if I want to meet at Target. Not even that could provide the desired distraction. How much more underwear and printed T-shirts do I need? I am tired of these trips and its connection to my chemotherapy.

There is additional agitation stirring within me. I don't feel prepared to be cured or in remission. More lessons must be rooted. Over the past seven months I've shown little external side effects. How can I really be dying if I still present as healthy? It's like everyone is going through the motions to cure this hidden beast and I still feel the urge to ask at every appointment, "You're sure this is cancer, right?"

Taking my seat in the Johns Hopkins imaging center, I chug the berry-flavored barium. Two hours after the dye contrast has fully coated my interior, a nurse inserts an IV. She struggles with the oversized latex gloves while complaining about Johns Hopkins' inadequate inventory and organization.

Just before the technician inserts me into the tire, I playfully ask him if he knows what parts of my body to photograph.

"So you're going to do the abdomen, pelvic, chest, and neck, riiight?"

He looks quizzically at his computer.

"No, we're doing the pelvic, abdomen, and chest."

What follows is a repetition of expletives. "I'm not getting off this table until my fucking neck is scanned," I scold. "I have a large mass on my jugular. What do you mean it wasn't ordered?!"

"Dr. Abbot didn't order it," the technician says flatly. The technician leaves me on the table to make the necessary calls. Meanwhile I ask his assistant to retrieve my cell phone from my bag. I ring my nurse navigator to report this fiasco. She's sweet and I know there is probably little she can do, but I expect more than, "You can call anytime you need to vent."

Ten minutes later, still lying in the machine with my pants down around my ankles, the technician comes back and adds my neck to his list of scans. Glad I was paying attention!

That night I seethe with anger for all those people who haven't advocated for themselves. How many patients have been killed by simple mistakes in hospitals, how many surgeries have been botched? We rely on these professionals to know our cases, to be in charge of our care. Patients must have a PhD in their illness to advocate for themselves. I was just being silly when I found their mistake, but I learned a valuable lesson: it would have been an inconvenience for me to take the additional CT scan the next day and I don't need inconveniences.

* * *

Having undergone the proper gamut of scans, I meet with Dr. Abbot by myself the next day. I want to receive news without worrying about my family's reactions. My mother and sisters gather in the waiting room as if I was in labor, waiting for the doctor to come out and declare, "It's a boy."

Dr. Abbot enters the room, hands me my printed results, and says, "Things look better, but there is a lot on there that the radiologist is describing in terms of lymph nodes so we want to do a PET scan to see if these things light up." She describes what the PET scan does and to this day I am still confused about which scan is desired. Dr. Abbot ushers me out of the office and into a blood draw room. Touching my shoulder as she turns to go, she says, "I'm so sorry."

* * *

Two minutes of gripping the foam vinyl padding of the armrests is all I can bear. There is one nurse attending to an elderly man down the hall. I pace in front of them. My mother and sisters have now been anticipating my news for forty-five minutes. I am working myself up into a tizzy on their behalf. Looking at the older gentleman down the hall getting all the attention, I think: *He's lived a full life, shouldn't I take precedence? Make him wait. I'm a middle-aged woman who hasn't seen her child go through puberty, celebrated her golden anniversary, or met her grandchildren. I'm running out of time, time that could be spent with my family right now if you just came and took my blood.* I catch my breath; how shameful I sound. Two nurses appear after my pacing becomes obnoxious. "Is everything okay?" one of them asks.

"No goddamnit!" I thump both armrests with each word. "I want my blood drawn now, so I can go out there and tell my family I still have cancer."

I push the doors open and step into the waiting room where my family sits with expectant anticipation. They turn to me as I enter. I shake my head. We huddle together as I give them my interpretation of the meeting. It is a blow. Nobody knows what to do or say except my mom, who says, "She's the same Beth she was a day ago."

As I leave my family to make an appointment for a PET scan, they follow me. I am really done with all of this, ALL of it. "Get out!" I yell at Jill, who is acting as my bodyguard, ready to pounce on whoever is making my life hell. She is protecting me and I berated her, for what? Not only am I confused about this other scan, I am mortified and sorry I hollered at Jill. Did I play up my reaction to Dr. Abbot and the need for a PET scan when I could have been calmer? If I'd had someone in the room with me they might have heard it differently. Perhaps the cancer is smaller, they need a PET scan to see what lights up and go from there. Jill was merely having a reflex to my own negative spin on things.

The nurse hands me preparations for the PET scan. Remain quiet, relaxed, and avoid stress for twenty-four hours prior to your exam. Too late for that, my appointment is in twelve.

The instructions to maintain a relaxed state make me particularly irritable. Since I am overwhelmed, I blame my mom and Jill for being overly sensitive to my feelings. No one can call it like it is, because my feelings about what it actually is are buried way down inside me. I accuse them of trying too hard not to annoy me, therefore annoying me. All I really want is to be alone, but I do not know how to say it. Instead I snap like a dog defending its food. It is eleven o'clock in the morning and I never drink before 5 p.m., but I sure am thinking about it. I call Todd to tell him I won't be home tomorrow, and for Noah not to call me tonight, because I will be busy trying to black out the events of the day.

Mom and Jill leave me at Karyn's house without the game of Bananagrams and the takeout sushi I promised them we would eat. Karyn and I share a bottle of wine; okay, a bottle and a half. Karyn drinks the half. Steadily we drink, except for a brief intermission when I call my therapist to ask existential questions. My incoherent babble doesn't render much advice so I return to the kitchen to continue my bender.

I settle back at the table, drink another glass of wine, and wonder how my blood alcohol level might affect tomorrow's PET scan. I know to avoid sugar and eat a high-protein diet, but the instructions said nothing about alcohol. Did they expect me to use my common sense? I keep my worry to myself. If I raise the question to my sister she might cut me off or feel guilty for supplying the wine. The day stressed her too and I imagine her cravings for a drink began as soon as I walked through those doors shaking my head.

After the wine, I share my uneasiness with Karyn. She goes straight to the internet and debunks my concern. Nonetheless, I spend a sleepless nervous night. I am ashamed by my debauchery.

* * *

The PET scan technician is a tall, sturdy man who instills me with confidence. I confess about drinking the night before. He laughs and assures me it will not have an effect.

He leaves me in the pitch dark, no reading, music, or phone usage allowed while I wait a full hour to reach a Zen state and the radioactive substance is fully absorbed. Now I am ready to be put into the pod.

After an hour in complete stillness, I dress and wait for the technician to write a note for me to hand to the security personnel and law enforcement officers at the airport. The note explains why I set off the security alarms and why I am nuclear. He proceeds to tell me to stay away from pregnant women, small children, and pets for at least eight hours.

Later that day I fly home and Todd picks me up from the airport. Dr. Kohler calls me with the PET scan results while we are driving: "There are areas on the PET scan that could either be cancer or postoperative changes. There are two things you can do. Nothing and get another scan in three months, or start a secondary chemotherapy treatment using different drugs."

"Are you saying I'm cured?" I asked him.

"Whoa, I'm not saying that. I'm saying there is cancer we can't detect."

I am so confused I have to ask him to call me later. He

wants me to come in for a face-to-face appointment to talk. At this point we both know I am not coming back. We agree to talk later that day, when he has more time.

That night, my phone rings. "Hello, Ms. Cramer. This is Dr. Kohler." Am I hearing the sound of scotch being poured over ice cubes? Is that the squeak of leather as he settles into his club chair? I picture Dr. Kohler alone in his study, taking off his tie, holding a cigar in one hand, and his drink in the other. His voice is as smooth as the good scotch he is drinking, which has already done its work of separating day from night. He has morphed back into a human being.

Dr. Kohler drops the medical jargon and asks me to do the same. He will not explain the differences between a CT scan and PET scan except to tell me the PET is more expensive and used only as a last resort. It doesn't matter to me anymore, he's drinking scotch, I'm having a glass of wine, and we are two friends in front of a crackling fire talking the truth. "If it were me?" he says, "I'd want to have quality of life. I'd live as well as I could until the end." I knew I would be having that face-to-face with Dr. Kohler after all. He became my hero in that one personal exchange.

Dr. Kan, my surgeon, also called me that night. When I ask him to explain why the CT scan and PET scan tell two different stories, he hedges, which tells me my question is not all that relevant. He reminds me that I have just finished a very strenuous first line of therapy. He does not mention next steps. I ask, "Am I in remission?"

He hesitates. "You could call it that." Sensing I am trying to give his words meaning, he offers, "You have been through a lot. My suggestion would be to take a break and enjoy your time with your son." I must be dying, I tell myself.

42

PASSOVER

April 20, 2018

We chop apples, nuts, and dried figs, pour Manischewitz into the mixture, and declare it the mortar Israelites used to build clay bricks when they were slaves in Egypt. My mom purchases fifteen quarts of matzah ball soup—seven more than we need and the Venetian spritzer is selected as the house cocktail. Enough wine is stocked to ensure every Jew can have at least four glasses, the seder plate is made, the table set, and fifteen Haggadahs placed on each seat: done. Except no one has prepared a service.

Todd, Noah, and I came to visit my family over spring break, which luckily falls on Passover. Though I'm not religious, the Jewish holidays have conditioned me to find my tribe and declare my ethnicity at least twice a year. Even a

Yankees fan has more pride than that. So I did not expect a wave of panic to come over me when I realized there was no one to lead our seder.

When I was a kid only men led the seder. It was always held at my grandmother's house: a matriarchal society except on Yom Kippur and Passover. Even then I felt uneasy about the gender roles at the table. My father always looked so pious and we were terrified to read the four questions from the Haggadah written in what looked like ancient text. My grandmother raised two boys, two girls, and had ten granddaughters. Women ruled under my grandmother's gentle and wise reign. I have to believe the main character who liberated the Israelites from Egypt wasn't Moses, but several brave women like my grandmother who orchestrated the whole thing. I bet Pharaoh was scared shitless of those feminists. She should have been leading us. But it is a nerve-racking responsibility to guide over twenty-five people spilling out of the dining room and into the entry hall. The ten granddaughters were practically seated in the pantry.

That experience was mine, not Noah's or Todd's, but I wanted it to be shared. Not because I want to start going to services or observe Shabbat, but because it is a memory of which I have few. It's a Hebrew memory bank that's augmented over time. The songs my sisters, cousins, and many of the people I have no other link to—but a similar history— have the same memory. We sing prayers boldly, not knowing the meaning. It's in our blood. I want it to be in Noah's.

He's not Jewish enough. It's my fault. We had pancakes for breakfast the first day of Passover. It never once occurred to me to stay away from bread. If you are gluten-free this is your holiday, but we exist on bagels and cream cheese.

* * *

I have thirty minutes until all the guests arrive to right this. Conveniently I brought my laptop. I take to the internet and type: child Haggadah. Passover told simply. Symbols of the seder plate. The story of Passover told in under fifteen minutes. Anything but the unabridged Passover Haggadah from the eighth century we have on hand, the same ones our great-great-grandparents read from.

This is not the first time I've been in this position. When we don't get together with family and find ourselves without plans for Passover, we scramble to pull one together at last minute. This is after we call anyone we know in our neighborhood with a somewhat Jewish last name and ask if they have a seat at their table. With four hours before a seder typically commences, inevitably a handful of stray Jews gravitate together.

Someone finds a drumstick in his or her freezer, another raids the neighbor's hen house for an egg, Todd goes to ShopRite and splits a box of matzah with a random woman in the same situation. No parsley? Onion grass will do. The only thing we have on stock is plenty of wine. A holiday that demands you drink at least four glasses over dinner is easily observed amongst our friends.

Here we are in Maryland, this seder has been thought out, brisket has been made well in advance, and we are just going to wing it? When the guests arrive at Mauri's, I am hunched over the computer. I feel like I've been assigned a news story that's due in ten minutes. "I'm sorry," I say to arrivals I haven't seen in months. "I'm just putting together a seder—real quick." Their faces tighten as one tells me about the long seder they attended the night before; the first night. Oh no, clearly they are not expecting anything ceremonial. I cut out the part where I was going to identify everything on the seder plate.

Once we all take our seats, I slug back whatever's left of my Venetian spritzer. Being at the head of the table where I am positioned, I could have easily had two glasses, but I missed cocktail hour because I allowed my inner geek to come out.

I start with a joke. "On this night Jews recline on a pillow in celebration of being free from slavery and enjoying well-deserved leisure time. Luckily they decided to lie on one side so they wouldn't choke to death defeating the whole purpose of survival. Anyways, my only reason for using a cushion tonight is to prop myself up so I can see over the table." That went over pretty well. I'm glad to be sober.

Down several seats from me I see Noah, the only youth under the age of twenty-two at the table. What I say next is off script. "The reason I wanted to have some kind of structure for our seder is because I am inspired by my son. I didn't realize how important it is to me to have Noah immersed in the same traditions we all grew up with. We don't even know how we know the rituals of this holiday or most of the Jewish holidays, because we weren't forced to. Our parents fed it to us and we are glad because we can sit around the table together and feel connected to one another. So I'll keep this short, but it's really important that my son grows up with the same recording we all have in our heads."

And I jumped in.

* * *

It went so well my sisters kept a copy for next year. All the guests, even my father, congratulated me. They enjoyed the fresh material. I felt like a Jewish warrior, one of the courageous women who led her people from slavery—or the lengthy seders we remember from our youth. I'm already thinking of next year and wondering if my family would be up for some group discussion about how the Passover story is relevant today.

Why is this Passover relevant to my own cancer story? I want to know. A year ago I doubt I would have had this passion and if so I wouldn't speak it. Am I letting my voice be heard, the one I didn't know I had? It is deeper than that though. My fear is that I won't pass down enough experiences to Noah. By retelling my experience of being Jewish, can I make him nostalgic for it? I fear him losing a part of me, something that may be of importance yet not be repeated.

43

SOMETHING LIKE REMISSION

June 12, 2018

For three months I decide I will do nothing that is punitive as I take to heart Dr. Kan's words: "Enjoy your time." If I see a food truck I stop. I'm tempted to eat a corn dog, not knowing what the hell it is. Suddenly I forget I am lactose intolerant and up until today have not eaten hot dogs as a rule. But now I am heading back to Johns Hopkins for my next scan. The prior scan we considered the scan of all scans? It wasn't, this one is.

Now that my white blood cells are not compromised I prepare to take the bus to DC instead of flying. I'm actually looking forward to this seven-hour trip. A few days prior to my departure Todd surprises me. He is going to drive me to

DC, but not only that, he booked a romantic boutique hotel in the heart of Georgetown and has made arrangements for the kids. This is thoughtfully planned out. I try to keep my mouth from gaping open as I chew on this terrible idea. Right after a CT scan is not an ideal time for a tryst. The look on Todd's face as he shares the surprise is so satisfied and precious. He is trying to please me and I want to do this for him. Besides, I have been waiting a long time for a romantic get away with my husband; my hair is growing back so maybe passion will as well. Grooming is in order and of course the facial hair has come back. It doesn't feel right to complain. Where hair has grown back in unwelcome places, I hesitate tweezing or shaving. I actually feel guilt when I do.

Others just see the stubble of hair on my head coming in like a five o'clock shadow. Todd tells me I look like a rock star. My friends tell me I look like a bad ass. I think I still look like an eighty-six-year-old Jewish man from Philadelphia.

My CT scan at four o'clock in the afternoon is going to leave me toxic for about forty-eight hours. I'll have to drink gallons of water, not wine, to eliminate the contrast dye I ingest. Cramping, diarrhea or constipation, and an outside chance of ringing in my ears, sweating, weakness, and confusion are expected. I hope for the best, give Todd a hug, and call my sister to gripe.

Ultimately, even if we stay in bed and order in dinner while watching TV, it will be ideal. By making this feel like a getaway instead of a hospital trip, Todd has put a positive spin on the purpose and possible outcome of our visit.

We have a fantastic time. I do have some stomach issues, but they subside quickly enough and don't get in the way of our night. The hotel provides. There is intimacy, honesty, and some shopping the next day before my appointment. Am I being set up to swallow some bad news or is this connection with Todd about to shift the tide?

We enter Johns Hopkins at 2 p.m. It is strange how unfamiliar Todd is with the hospital layout, having been here only one other time in the past nine months. It occurs to me that Todd has not insisted on coming and I have not invited him. It is as if I fear his vision of me getting an infusion or a scan will poison our "healthy" relationship. So I spare him those gloomy events. Todd's living with my hair loss was enough of a reminder that he might lose me. While I know Todd is stoic and loyal, I have not trusted him completely.

* * *

As we sit in the waiting room I harbor fears of new cancer growth I did nothing to avoid. I pull out the three-ring binder I have been filling with all my cancer information since diagnosis and turn to the nutrition page. I confess that I have not followed a single one of the recommendations on the diet. No gluten? I ate plenty. No dairy? I found a new love for ice cream. I guiltily go down the list pointing out all the vegetables, protein, fats, and herbs I was warned not to eat. I'm screwed.

Stage 4 cancer does not get cured, it is a terminal illness and it has helped me to say, "fuck it" more. At dinner with a good friend a few weeks ago, I expounded on the merits of cancer as a gift. Midsentence, I paused. It sounded like I was recommending a great book. I told my friend, "I'm sorry, I hear myself twisting my situation to sound favorable.

You do not need a life-threatening event to change who you are or your perspective."

* * *

Dr. Kohler begins with twenty questions about my health.

"How is your appetite?"

"Fine."

"Energy?"

"Fine."

"Neuropathy?"

"Fine." Todd and I sense he is leading up to drop a bomb.

Finally he says, "So the scan was good. The bottom line is further improvement since the previous study. I would be in no hurry to get treatment. They are getting smaller without treatment."

"Is that what you call remission?" Todd asks.

"I think it's pretty darn close. At this point I think we can just watch. What would you like to do?"

He is asking me?

"We'll see you back here in three months as long as you're feeling well. I don't think anyone thinks this is the last page in the story, unfortunately, because you had pretty extensive disease to start. At the moment there's nothing active, which doesn't mean there is nothing at all. Probably there, but asleep."

"I can't believe I haven't done anything wrong in the last three months to wake them up." I'm fishing.

"Which is good. So whatever you're doing, keep doing it."

I slowly turn my head toward Todd with an incredulous look. We simultaneously shrug in a gesture of disbelief and chuckle. "Really? Okay."

I heard Dr. Kohler say it's far from over, but if I keep living my way, without restriction, who's to know? The timeline is working out nicely. Tom came in September when I was diagnosed and now he is returning to Paris when I am somewhere close to remission. Rereading a letter he wrote me in May when I was traveling back and forth to DC, I am amazed and flattered by his observation. He wrote, *I want to thank you for all you do for me. It's amazing to be with you, to live with you. You are the strongest woman I know. Even during bad times you know how to react and solve the problems.*

My cancer journey must be over (for now), since it is his time to go. I can imagine him reading the letter I wrote him over the Atlantic:

Dear Tom,

When you arrived I knew an angel had been sent to help me and my family through what could have been a very difficult time. Your smile has lit up this house and has never stopped shining. I am so very proud of you, Tom. At fifteen you came to America, with difficulty understanding English, and at sixteen you leave a fluent speaker. You have made incredible choices that are advanced for your years. Leaving your home and entering a different culture, opening yourself up to experiences you couldn't anticipate was the bravest thing I can imagine doing. This experience has set you up for a big life. We all will forever keep our doors open for you.

Love, Beth

* * *

I am not wasting time. I have new dreams to fulfill, but our personal accounts are not going to support them. So, I make an early withdrawal from my IRA. There really should be an exception for terminally ill patients whose life expectancy has shortened to use it without tax penalty. Yesterday, I bought myself a pre-owned Audi TT convertible. Before buying it I underplayed how much I wanted it, assuring Todd that I am fully aware that external things don't bring inner peace. Truthfully, every time I get in that car and put the top down, it is a vacation.

I enroll Todd, Noah, and myself in scuba diving training to become PADI certified so we can discover the last frontier under water, and then I book a week of diving in the Dutch Caribbean. Call me overconfident, but I plan an expedition to South Africa and pay for it eight months in advance with no trip insurance. It is nonrefundable.

44

LAST ONE STANDING

There were four women in our small college town: a visual artist, a life coach, a yoga instructor, and a healer. It didn't matter to cancer that they were health conscious, conservationists, mothers, and under fifty-five. I came to rely on these women as role models for how I should live my life years before they were diagnosed. They were self-possessed women with desires and strength to overcome adversity. I wanted what they were having. Therefore, at different points I employed their individual talents to heal me of my second-child dilemma.

Lili led her life chasing adventure. She radiated determination and confidence. Lili had a business degree, was an accomplished photographer following world-class skiers off cliffs, made many films, and was a conservationist. It was not until her late forties that she had her two children and went back to college to earn an MFA in printmaking. The calligraphy hanging on her studio door says *this is it*, from Thich Nhat Hanh.

Lili and I both moved from New York City to New Paltz the same summer and met at our children's kindergarten orientation. We were both filmmakers and laughed that we would enroll our children in a no-technology school that bans screen time. Lili had known me as an ambitious and somewhat competitive person who wanted it all. But after my fire went out she scolded me. "What happened? When I met you, you were this powerhouse. You were driven." She thought I was one of her own. I no longer cared about my career; she had won the ultimate prize of mothering two. Her perspective is that if you want something, you do it. Lili didn't only decide to become a mother late in life; she elected to adopt two children whose birth mothers were addicted to drugs. After every walk with Lili, I would feel the courage to get pregnant or start the adoption process I was so obsessed with. She joked that she would be after me if I didn't go through with it. Lili passed away from brain cancer in December of 2015.

Elizabeth had adopted four children, two from Guatemala and two from Rwanda, forming a small united nations. She enrolled all of them in the Mountain Laurel Waldorf School, where my son and Lili's daughter attended. Elizabeth was an Amazon compared to me in many ways. She was a six-foot-tall extrovert who always looked like she was ready to tackle at the line of scrimmage: head down and bent at the waist, ready to rush whatever was ahead of her. I'd see her wide-mouthed smile from across the parking lot. There she is, I would think, chaos and laughter all bundled into one.

Elizabeth was the self-proclaimed adoption goddess, and had a business guiding clients through the arduous adoption process, both logistically and emotionally. I became Elizabeth's client. Her goal was to have me make an inspired action plan toward fulfilling my dream of parenting again. It was to be a five-month process from the time we started working together to the moment I was on my way via pregnancy or adoption. At month five I was still working exercises from month three, and she was mentoring me twice a week. My movie masterpiece, as she called it, was still in development with no sign of coming to the screen.

Our hours of walking meditations, visualizations, and creating an altar of random charms for my sacred space were pretty hilarious. As much as I prayed Elizabeth's karma would rub off on me, I was Teflon. She adopted four kids. My heart wanted one more, but my anxiety stomped all over that notion.

Just as I was getting close to choosing my path, when I needed one final push, Elizabeth canceled our session. I didn't hear from her for weeks. A text came letting me know she had become sick, with cancer. This was not the time to ask for a pep talk.

Growing up, illness had a smell. If I saw someone sick I'd go the other way. When I was a kid my best friend at camp fainted in my presence and I avoided her the rest of the summer. Visiting a hospital, I would hold my nose until I left. I still do sometimes. Since I'd had some practice nursing Lili, I was more confident in my ability to care for people. When Elizabeth asked me to drive her to chemotherapy, I didn't think twice. Elizabeth was the one I was driving to chemotherapy when I got pulled over by a police officer. Before the cop could say license and registration, I blurted, "My friend is late for her chemotherapy, and it's my fault." As I've said, he escorted us to the entrance. The rest of Elizabeth's and my day together turned into a situational comedy. I was easing up on disease, and it felt good to discover this part of myself.

A year later Elizabeth went into remission. It didn't take long for her to jump into a new venture: life coaching. She offered me free counseling as a practice client, which she needed for earning a certification. I declined, but her path was cut short anyway. The chemotherapy-induced leukemia was the last straw.

Prior to her funeral, Elizabeth's husband asked me to create a video using various photographs of her fifty-four years put to songs she had written and performed. It was shown at the memorial service. I remember seeing Erica Chase-Salerno, another local living with cancer, sitting four rows back with her two young children flanking her. It occurred to me that the same people at Elizabeth's memorial would be attending Erica's. I wondered what she was thinking. Was she imagining her own memorial? Would I have brought Noah to this funeral if I were in her shoes? Were Erica's children imagining their own mother's smiling face projected on the screen, their memories playing out in a nicely edited video? It was surreal and heartbreaking to imagine Erica next in line.

Erica Chase-Salerno. Erica was mythical, a social star in the Hudson Valley. I met Erica in the playground when I first moved to town. She was feverishly posting the moments of her life on Facebook. Clearly Erica was busy befriending everyone around her, because she started a conversation with me. I learned her obsession with Facebook was not trite; it was a way for her to create the human chain. This was a platform for her to spread positivity and information with inspiration on where to find it. Erica was serious about getting others to find their truth.

Erica was a skilled spiritual healer. Wylde Acres, her professional practice, according to her website offered "private holistic pregnancy and general healing sessions to help mothers connect more deeply with their babies, as well as their innermost selves. By hearing what your own spirit is saying, I can help you clear away some mental fog, indecision, anguish, and help you connect with your personal truths." She was the perfect counselor for me. Indecision and anguish all centered on reproduction? I was pulled to her like a magnet. I could have poured my heart out in her presence even though I had only met her a handful of times. I am certain two thousand of her Facebook followers felt the same way.

The week after my acute breakdown, I found Erica on the soccer field. Our children weren't on the same team, but it was easy to spot her two fields away. Erica sparkled. Her oversized thick-rimmed sunglasses, large bright red costume jewelry, cowboy boots, and crazy hat were nothing compared to the personality balancing all those elements. If she wasn't engaged in a passionate conversation with someone, Erica looked like she had been completely taken by surprise by a magnificent gift. I had never met anyone so animated.

The day Erica and I spoke on the sports field, I was looking for counsel. She didn't want me as a client though. She wanted me to forgive myself and be grateful that I did not have that baby. "Clearly it wasn't meant to be or it would have happened," she told me. It was that simple in Erica's opinion. There are no accidents. There were no answers to seek.

Erica lived with cancer for four years. Her journey became a social phenomenon. She was proud to be the poster child of cancer. Besides posting pictures of herself on Facebook with tubes linked to her veins, revealing the latest rash or scar from a brain incision, Erica wrote a weekly column in the local newspaper: "Erica's Cancer Journey."

When I told Erica I had cancer, the ironic connection between my baby crisis and my ovarian cancer was not lost on her. Right away I tried to use my misfortune as a creative project, curious if it could fuel a documentary. With no direction established, I rushed to interview Erica with hopes that it would spur an idea.

Suffering from dizziness from my chemotherapy regimen, I arrived at Erica's house and unloaded my video equipment. I arranged Erica in a chair, had her wear an outfit that was not too colorful, and redecorated the wall behind her to eliminate any distraction. I made sure to make use of any natural light. I was awkwardly mindful of her time even though she loved this opportunity. I snaked the wireless microphone up her shirt and she was ready to go, no trepidation or apology. She thanked me and complimented my craft, making sure I knew how much she respected and trusted my artistry and genius. Erica was everyone's cheerleader. All I had to do was point the camera at her and push record. I was aware that so many things could go wrong even doing a small shoot like this: the focus could be soft or I might record crappy audio or run out of storage with no backup. Erica's possible expectations for this video suddenly took on an importance I hadn't considered. It would be going in her legacy box.

The first question I asked was broad. "What do you want me to know?" An hour and a half later, I had a chance to ask a follow-up question. There was none. She was poised, never lost her train of thought, brought up one aspect after another, and it was enlightening. But I wasn't truly listening. I was too busy being self-involved, waiting for the nugget that would distinguish my documentary. I started to wish I could stop her and ask pointed questions. She was having a very deep, personal conversation with not just her fan base, but humanity. When I left I knew I would never use it, there would be no documentary.

Erica never got to see the finished product. I never edited it together; truthfully I never even watched it through. The idea of making a documentary was fraught with negatives. I was going to live my movie; dedicating my career to it would be grueling. I transferred the media to my drives, expecting to never visit it again. What was I going to tell Erica? If I solely put the raw footage on a disc and handed it to her, it would seem crass, like I didn't think her message was important. I told myself she would forget about it since she had already been interviewed on radio and in print, and her story was all over social media. My video was inconsequential. I did what every normal person does; I avoided it.

When I saw Erica she never brought up the interview, not even to ask how it looked. Erica would never put pressure on another person and I am sure she accepted that I was going through my own shit.

The day after Erica passed I couldn't sleep, thinking about the media on my hard drive. At 3 a.m. I got out of bed, went to my office, and watched Erica, looking directly into camera, telling me about all the wonderful insights cancer had brought her. It was one and a half years since the day I'd interviewed her. I was one and a half years into my own cancer journey and I was ready to listen. I posted her video on Facebook the following morning. Boy was I glad I'd had her look directly into the camera. We both knew that preserving her image in this way would make it into her legacy box and again she was reminding me to start filling my own. Erica passed February 7, 2019.

Angela. Angela died two days before Erica. She moved back to England, her birthplace, and spent her final year there. We emailed back and forth sharing our war stories. Angela chose to take the holistic route, as opposed to Erica's cocktail of chemo, radiation, surgeries, etc. Angela took being health conscious very seriously. She was vegan, taught yoga every day, and was close to finishing her master's degree in nutrition. When Angela and I got talking at any party, and after I had glass of wine, she'd have me 90 percent committed to doing a colon cleanse.

Angela flittered around New Paltz like an angel, just as her name suggests. Her beautiful son, who shared her blond hair, blue eyes, and lithe frame, went to the Mountain Laurel Waldorf School with my son, Lili's daughter, and Elizabeth's four kids. We would see Angela, her son and her husband (literally the yoga guru of our town) at least once a month when a few Jewish families gathered for a Shabbat potluck and conversation.

Angela's family would arrive at these gatherings looking like they just stepped out of *Om Yoga Magazine*. They walked through the world with such mindfulness it seemed almost naïve. We made fun of how much food Angela could consume at our potlucks. She would enter with a small kale salad and leave with containers of leftovers. Her son was a picky eater, but that didn't stop her from preparing overloaded plates and setting them aside with a sticky note warning "DO NOT DISCARD." The only time I saw Angela look at all confrontational was when someone got close to her son's plate.

It was shocking to find out cancer had come for Angela. Her plans did not include illness and invasive therapies. She was about to be a certified clinical nutritionist. Last I saw her she was practically skipping around town gathering clients. I was high up on her list.

Seems like quite a cluster. I'm not sure what they might link it to, yoga, writing, me? We are a cluster of women who had monikers like *goddess, head on heart strong, maverick,* and my own *brave.* When these women passed they had a lot on their plates and were still filling it with more, even after cancer ended up on the buffet.

The women are all gone now. Their obituaries have been taken off the funeral home's server. Erica's article chronicling her life no longer appears in the newspaper we receive every Thursday. I wonder how their families live, how their lives have changed? Are they relieved to be free of watching their mother and wives fade? Did they know life would go on? Are they surprised that it already has?

Some days I feel it's coming for me. The cancer. It's just a matter of time. I am the last one standing.

45

SHEMA

Soon after my diagnosis, I started to imagine all the people I would see in the afterlife. Why not? There would be the child I gave up. My grandmother, Nathlie, would be expecting me: the first of ten granddaughters to join her in the afterlife. I wonder if there are scooped oranges and waffles in heaven. Mr. McDowell, my elementary school's janitor and my confidant, who I followed around the halls pushing a broom just to be near him, would save me a seat in Heaven's cafeteria. My childhood dog, Bonnie, who I always knew was god spelled backward would be at my side.

My last eight years have been very busy chasing clarity. It did not come from a yoga retreat or sitting on top of Machu Picchu with a monk. My version of clarity was suspect as it depended on making choices. Todd likes to remind me, "No matter where you go, there you are."

Perspective arrived with cancer. This disease rose up and swallowed my incessant yakking.

* * *

I'm heading to Kripalu, a center for yoga and health in Massachusetts, for a few days of R&R alone. I sit on our screened porch, my hair wet from a swim, when Todd walks in with dirt and grass clippings stuck to his face and beads of sweat glimmering on his brow. He wipes his oily hands on a cloth in such a way that I know he is feeling put out.

"You're mad at me. What's wrong? It's that I'm going away, isn't it?"

"What exactly do you need a break from?" he asks as if he had been ruminating on this during every lap of the yard he mowed.

"I can't do the work I need to do here; I need time alone. I feel like I've been babysat the last nine months. I want to reconnect with myself. You think this has been one long vacation for me, don't you?"

"No, but I don't think what you are looking for can be bought or found a hundred miles away."

"Right, wherever you go…"

"…there you are. Yes," Todd finishes.

"Actually I've heard the phrase can be attributed to Confucius who actually said, 'Wherever you go, go with all your heart.'"

"That is not what this trip is about. You've said yourself you're not sure why you're going," Todd says.

"That's because you don't understand what I am looking for."

"I guess I don't."

"Because you're not interested in looking inward yourself. Having new experiences actually takes leaving the house."

An hour later I pick up my weekend bag and start for the door only to dodge a bat. This is terrifying, but then I remember a night in 2012 when my mind was looping around my decision to use an egg donor. I had called my therapist. While on the phone a bat flew in circles like it was making rotations around the sun. My therapist immediately looked up the symbolism of bats. "Bats sleep in caves or dark places. This is symbolic of the womb. The bat is a symbol of rebirth and it is a creature that lives in the belly of the mother." I interpreted this one way: that a baby wanted to come and no matter how much fear I had around it, it was my mission to conceive. I was not ready to consider any other meaning. That bat visited me every night for the next three.

A bat hasn't visited me again until today. I leave with the intent to reflect on my life and consider my rebirth. I looked up the symbolism again and found more: "The animal's position hanging upside down parallels that of the unborn self, immersed in darkness. Bat medicine is there to help you to let go of old habits and a previous way of life, and to face a new dawn…Face your fears. Be flexible. Prepare for rebirth. The time is now, the power is yours."

I never considered myself a witch, but I'm starting to wonder. Bats do not just randomly appear in our house. There has to be some message. If before the bat was telling me to birth another child, now it is telling me to birth myself.

I put down the tennis racquet and bravely make my escape from the house. Still holding on to anger against

Todd I get into my car, start the engine, and begin to back out of the driveway. Magically my baby anthem song "A Thousand Years" comes through the speakers. No apps are turned on. Not iTunes, not Spotify, not Pandora. I swear it.

I have died every day waiting for you
Darling, don't be afraid I have loved you
For a thousand years
I'll love you for a thousand more.

I have intentionally avoided that song for almost as many years. Why did it play now and from where? What's next? Will I drive into a vortex that will lead to Heaven's Gate? No ending had been outlined for this story and it presents a surprising twist. Though I am not convinced it's a winner.

* * *

Arriving at Kripalu I can feel my excitement building with the perfect weather and the beauty of Stockbridge fueling it. The entrance winds up a private road with posted signs, Quiet Please. The sprawling lakefront campus is sweet, but the large brick building that was once a monastery screams institution.

I have registered for a shared room as a way to test my ability to face my fears and let go of old habits. When I get to the reception desk I remind myself that I am here to encourage transformative positive shifts. Oh hell, what am I doing taking a chance on being drawn into conversation by a snoring bunkmate? Even if I wore a sign pinned to my chest stating I am in silence, it would be distracting. I fork over my credit card for an upgrade to a single room and thank myself for being flexible just like the bat told me to be.

A friend told me to check out the spa and the excellent hot tub. Following the signs down to the boiler room I reserve judgment. Luxury is not the point of this retreat, but expectations die hard. All I ever hear about Kripalu is the incredible food. The wafting smell of an old-age home leads me to the cafeteria. The buffet of macrobiotic dishes brings the smell closer. The most disappointing aspect of this whole thing is that I am clearly not a truly spiritual person like all those who have made the pilgrimage here and I am missing the point of Kripalu!

I may not drink the Kripalu Kool-Aid, but I cannot go home with my tail between my legs. I want to call Todd and apologize; he too would have softened by now. I remind myself that he will be there for me when I get back with an apology of his own. I text "I love you" and get a heart back in return. Shutting my phone off again, I decide to take a walk in the woods and give myself a pep talk. I am here to reconnect with myself. I cannot let the external influences matter. It is not about the destination, it is about what I find along the way. I use the trail map to find an actual destination to hang my travel hammock. The trail heading to an old-growth forest is supposed to have dappled sunlight coming through the trees and solitude. Clutching onto this image, I am frustrated by the three loops I make around the red trail, but I refuse to give into anything less than what was promised. What an asshole, I can't even let go of the destination. Anyway, I start to head back to the Kripalu grounds.

Something I hear stops me in my tracks. I look up to the sky, checking for signs of angels. I identify strings and woodwinds…coming from a church maybe? It beckons me in the opposite direction of Kripalu. I leave the trail and hack my way out of the forest until I find myself standing in the middle of a country road. On the other side of the street is a manicured hedgerow. The music grows louder as I approach. Continuing the length of the shrubbery, I find an opening, turn the corner, and face a vast lawn leading to a shed, which I now recognize as Tanglewood. The Boston Symphony Orchestra is rehearsing for that night's performance, but at this moment it is just for me.

I make a bed for myself against a big oak and close my eyes. This is more than luck. An hour later they seem to be wrapping up, but instead a choir joins them. A large one. These enormous, breathtaking voices belt out one phrase so unexpected and familiar it takes my breath away. "Sh'ma Yisrael Adonai..." The soprano's voice singing in Hebrew stops my heart. This is a voice of unearthly beauty. It's the "Mourner's Kaddish." I know I haven't transitioned to the afterlife yet, but I trust that at this moment, I am exactly where I am supposed to be. If I did not have cancer I most likely would have missed it.

EPILOGUE

I was almost convinced I could sell an authentic happy Hollywood ending. Ultimately a terminal illness changed my relationship with time. Hear me scream it from a cliff on a magical isle: "Life matters!" The voice that says "you can't" has been buried. This is the stuff that makes for good resolution.

After the great news Todd and I heard from Dr. Kohler in June, I spent three more months fully living to survive per his advice, "Keep doing what you're doing." In anticipation of a full remission after my next CT scan in September, my sisters, mother, and I planned a trip to Colorado the very next day.

* * *

September 11, 2018: Mom, Karyn, and I squeeze into Dr. Kohler's examination room to hear the results from the scan I had the day before. I am so certain this meeting is going to be uneventful that I don't bother to record it. He asks the rudimentary questions, his eyes always hard to read. He feels around my neck and chest, rattles off a dimension to his nurse who inputs it into the computer, and I know. The lymph nodes are growing back. One is twice the size since it was last measured. I was two weeks shy of six months since my last chemotherapy, which classifies me as "platinum resistant." Platinum is the silverish metal I fondly wear around my neck and an element in my chemotherapy cocktail. My body likes platinum too much; it wasn't going to help fight my cancer.

Dr. Kohler saw my reluctance to aggressively dig back into treatment. "Ninety-eight percent of patients would go for treatment immediately, but studies show those who wait three months have the same life expectancy as those treated right away. Since you are asymptomatic you might want to wait," he says. Reading my mind, he continues, "You will know when you feel symptoms and you will want something to treat them." When Dr. Kohler leaves the room, my mom seems to melt into a cascade of tears. It is so surreal I think we are all characters in *The Isa Stories*. I have been living within those pages. We would get to the last chapter and put it down, pick up a lighter novel the next time. But the book isn't over:

Isa's mother trembles, her small sturdy frame now fragile from the years this one moment stole. Isa folds her mother into her arms awkwardly at first and says, "I am so sorry."

* * *

When I pushed Dr. Kan to tell me how long I had a year ago (worst-case scenario), I was just being dramatic, a scene for the book. I didn't actually think there would be a worst-case scenario. Two years. It has been one year almost to the day since that meeting, and what I find on the internet for life expectancy for platinum resistant ovarian cancer gives an average of twelve months. I believe I will well outlast that, but one thing is certain, I will always be living with cancer, different from living after cancer. As long as I keep controlling it with treatment it might not grow or even shrink, but it will never go away and stay away.

Things are changing in the ovarian cancer field and there is every reason to believe a new treatment will come along to expand my time. But for the first time I am overwhelmed with fear. Proof comes in the form of the travel insurance I purchased for my nonrefundable trip to South Africa in April.

Every time I turn a corner I wonder if what is happening is actually irony. I am now participating in a clinical trial made possible in part by Cycle for Survival donations. My family has started a team in Bethesda with Karyn as the captain. Karyn wrote a beautiful letter asking for support. The plight in her words was so true that any humorous retort I might give would fall flat.

Your gift will directly help people like Beth who have few, if any, treatment options.

I had been a marvel in my ability to be physically and mentally strong for one good year. It is now Thanksgiving, November 2018, and from where I sit on the back porch of our rented house in Curaçao, looking past our endless pool out to the turquoise ocean while Noah and Todd scuba dive, I thank cancer as much as I fear it. I had forgotten to seize the moments of my life. It shouldn't come at a price.

If you asked me today to rattle off ten reasons to live, I could give you details that fill an hour. I am not ready to die. I don't want to leave my family. Every day I take pride in my Noah and I am comforted by his bravery and skill. I am excited by my ability to provide opportunities for him. Will it be enough to cushion the fall of losing a mother? Yesterday he took his first night scuba dive; today I taught him to drive. Metaphorically I open the candy store to him whenever I can. My very dear Noah, always remember your strength, your goodness, and your incredible ability to make others uplifted. When I told myself I wanted more children, it was because you opened my heart in a way I never knew could have existed. That mission was a fool's errand. All I wanted was more of you and you have been here all along.

ACKNOWLEDGMENTS

To my sisters Mauri, Karyn and Jill: without you I wouldn't be a writer. You have given me so much material throughout our lives. I am so grateful we have eachother. Every moment along this path, I knew I could count on you telepathically. You are the reason this year looked easier than it should.

My mother has encouraged my endeavor to write from early on and hasn't stopped praising every email. There is no braver, more hopeful sparkling star on our planet. You are always the first person I cry to and I am thankful that you accept that as a compliment. Forever our leader, forever my anchor.

To my father, who although quiet in the background, is the loudest voice in my head. We are more alike than you will ever know. Without your example and confidence in me none of this would be possible.

I am grateful to have an incredible husband who has watched me day in and day out craft this story without asking, "What the hell are you still writing about?" Todd is an incredible caregiver, my best friend, and my partner in life.

Noah, I can only hope this book has in some way expressed how much I love you. Our bond is unearthly and therefore will exist forever. What a gift you have given me. Your humor, insight, and enthusiasm, along with your intensity and fury, have taught me so much about how to live.

You are on every page. You are my muse.

Some names, locations, and identifying characteristics have been changed to protect the privacy of those depicted. Dialogue has been re-created from memory.

My book is an accurate memoir of my life story, though I have changed some names.

Thank you to all my medical providers
Dr. Riolin Andrade, Hudson Valley Oncology
Dr Jeffrey Y. Lin, Director, Sibley Center for Gynecologic Oncology and Advanced Pelvic Surgery
Dr Bruce Kressel, medical oncologist at Johns Hopkins Kimmel Cancer Center at Sibley Memorial
Dr Pedro Ramirez, Gynecologic Oncologist at MD Anderson
Dr Rachel N. Grisham, Medical Oncologist at Sloan Kettering
Dr. David Hyman, Medical Oncologist at Sloan Kettering

Thanks to everyone on my publishing team, editors Carol Bergman and NaNá Stoelzle. A special thanks to Laura Boyle, the greatest cover designer, and Rachel Cone-Gorham, marketing expert.

ABOUT THE AUTHOR

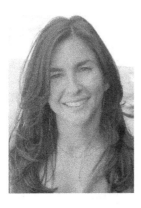

Beth Cramer is an accomplished editor and director of independent films, commercials and music videos. Her award-winning documentary "Plan B, Single Women Choosing Motherhood," explores the social picture single motherhood presents and why this trend is snowballing among women in their thirties and forties. In 2017 Cramer was diagnosed with stage IV ovarian cancer and her memoir, *Why Didn't I Notice Her Before?*, documents her experience as a mother, wife, sister and daughter through her diagnosis. Irreverent, painfully honest and often hilarious, *Why Didn't I Notice Her Before?* has a rhythm and pacing that makes it compulsively readable. Today, Cramer lives with her husband and son in the Hudson Valley and spends her time writing and creating.

CPSIA information can be obtained
at www.ICGtesting.com
Printed in the USA
LVHW111228250819
628859LV00002B/464/P